Praise for

YOU Rule! Take Charge of Your Health and Life

"I highly recommend this book! It is a great resource for providers to share with their patients to reinforce positive health behaviors."

—**Tonya Jefferson, DNP, FNP, APRN**
Founder and CEO of The Walkin Clinic

"I have to say…I love it! I want to promote it in middle schools and high schools! Thank you for your contribution; your research looks spot on. Great work!"

—**Cecile Martin-Jones**
FNP-BC, APRN, MS, RN
Sleep Medicine Program

"Being healthy has never been easy. Dr. Antwala makes it less painful for all concerned. If you are the parent of a teen, you should buy this book. If you are a teen, you should read this book."

—**Tasha Roberts**
Mompreneur and CEO
Hadiya Wellness

"If you're a teenager looking to improve your health, life, and success read YOU Rule immediately. It cuts straight to the chase on what you need to know to live healthy and thrive, and will impact your life enormously. A must-read for all youth who want to live healthy and be successful while doing it."

—**Kim Hardy**
Best-selling author of Relaunch
Kim Hardy Speaks

YOU Rule!
TAKE CHARGE OF YOUR HEALTH AND LIFE

A HEALTHY LIFESTYLE GUIDE FOR TEENS

Dr. Antwala Robinson

This book contains advice and information relating to health care. It should be used to supplement rather than replace the advice of your medical provider or another trained health professional. If you know or suspect that you have a health problem, it is recommended that you seek the advice of your medical provider before embarking on any medical program or treatment. All efforts have been made to ensure the accuracy of the information contained in this book as of the date of publication. The author disclaims liability for any medical outcomes that may occur as a result of applying the methods suggested in this book.

Copyright © 2014 by Antwala Robinson, DNP, FNP-C, APRN

All rights reserved. No portion of this book may be reproduced, stored in a retrieval system, or transmitted in any form or by any means - electronic, mechanical, photocopy, recording, scanning, or other - except for brief quotations embodied in critical reviews or articles.

Printed in the United States of America.

ISBN 978-0-9903748-0-0

This book may be purchased for educational, business, or sales promotional use. For information please contact: The Wellness Agent, 4480-H, South Cobb Drive, #491 Smyrna, GA 30080 or email us at info@thewellnessagent.com

The Wellness Agent website: www.thewellnessagent.com

This book is dedicated to

My daughter and to all youth around the world.
Know that you can live a healthy lifestyle and the life you dream of.
But you must have WHY POWER, because Will Power alone is
not enough. Determine your WHY, then let it be the FORCE
that drives you!

The loving memories of my parents and two sisters, who believed in
me and were my biggest cheerleaders. Your love still shines
through in all my endeavors.

All those who fight to save the lives of our youth, and help them
improve their health and overall quality of life while on their
quest to becoming productive individuals.

TABLE OF CONTENTS

INTRODUCTION 11

CHAPTER 1

Health and Wellness 13

Healthy Diet and Healthy Weight 13
Unhealthy Eating Habits 22
Healthy and Unhealthy Fats 29
Water 33
Physical Activity and Exercise 36
Immune System 47
Sleep 50

CHAPTER 2

Physical Health 55

Annual Physical Examinations 55
Eye Health 56
Dental Health 58

CHAPTER 3 60

Reproductive Health 60

Female Puberty 60
Male Puberty 66
Personal Hygiene 69
Infertility 70
Teenage Pregnancy 72
HIV (Human Immunodeficiency Virus) 74

Contraceptives and Birth Control Methods 78
Abstinence 82

CHAPTER 4
Common Chronic Diseases in Youth 86

Common Chronic Diseases in Youth 86
Obesity 88
Asthma 93
Type 1 Diabetes (Juvenile Diabetes) 97
Acne 100

CHAPTER 5
Building Relationships 105

Communication – the pillar of strong relationships 106
Family Relationships 108
Building Healthy Friendships 111
Sexual Orientation – LGBT (Lesbian, Gay, Bisexual, and Transgender) 113

CHAPTER 6
Teen Social Media Relationships and Privacy 122

Sharing Personal Information 124
Having a Healthy Social Media Presence 126
Maintaining Healthy Social Media Relationships 129

CHAPTER 7
Unhealthy Relationships 132

Dating Violence 136
Bullying and Peer Pressure 139

CHAPTER 8

Developing Character 143
    Respect 145
    Responsibility 146

CHAPTER 9

Your Mental and Emotional Health 152
    Your Mental and Emotional Health 153
    Mental and Emotional Disorders 156
    Substance Abuse 158
    Tobacco Use 164
    Alcohol Abuse 173
    Teen Suicide 180
    Community Service 186
    Meditation 187
    Principles for Success 189

CHAPTER 10

Rights as a Teen when Seeking Healthcare 199

CONCLUSION 204

RESOURCES 205

REFERENCES 217

INDEX 224

ABOUT THE AUTHOR 227

INTRODUCTION

Adan's family moved to the United States 5 years ago from Spain when he was only 10. Call it a language barrier or his immigrant status, but; he always had to try pretty hard just to fit in, until he landed in high school. Fortunately, he got a chance to be a part of the "cool" group. But he is in a dilemma these days.

His parents don't like his friends and are always criticizing the "new habits" he has recently adopted (like smoking, drinking and wearing sagging pants). Adan is under so much pressure that he just doesn't know what to do. He has started to hate his parents, who he thinks are so old-fashioned and too conservative.

Natasha, a 16-year-old, has no immigrant issues like Adan, no language barrier and no "uncool habits," yet nobody at school wants to talk to her. Her classmates call her names like "geek," "weirdo," and "nerd." She often asks herself if being a smart and hardworking student is such a big deal. Having no friends, no boyfriends and nobody to talk to is now taking a toll on Natasha's health. She just doesn't know what to do.

Katie is an adorable girl, with blonde hair and green eyes. She is pretty popular in her school too. Two years ago, she chose Gary among hundreds of other guys who approached her. But it seems she made a wrong decision, as Gary is not only violent, but also has a tendency to frequently get jealous, agitated, and physical.

Katie tried explaining to him a few times that she is getting sick of his bipolar attitude, but Gary sure is a sweet talker when he needs to be. He has assured Katie that he loves her, but when she does "weird stuff" like giving more time to her studies or her other friends, he gets annoyed. He told her, "I just can't share you with anyone." Katie feels proud that Gary loves her so much, but also feels that his behavior is irrational most of the times.

Being a teenager is not easy. A lot of teens want the liberty to make decisions like an adult, but you should understand that adolescence has its own challenges and issues. Are you aware that:

- About 8% of adolescents seek medical treatment for major depression? Yet the overall prevalence of depression in teenagers is 28%; this means the remaining 20% battle with pressure and depression without any medical support.
- Suicide is among the tenth leading causes of death in the US adult population, but the second leading cause of death in adolescents.
- About 25% of all teens reported being abused by their dating partner via texts or phone; yet most teens tolerate the abuse like Katie and never report it. Most importantly, no intervention is taken in almost 90% of the cases as reported by the Urban Institute.

There are a number of other problems that teens face, yet the resources and help are mostly unavailable (or teens are uniformed as to where and how to seek the appropriate help).

Isn't it pretty alarming?

Healthcare providers believe that early resolution of issues in youth can prevent complications and extreme events later in life. This book examines the major issues facing youth today, and how they can "take charge" of their health and life to prevent and/or manage these issues and ultimately live a healthy lifestyle.

This book contains real stories that you may have read/ heard in news and forgotten about. The author has tried to explain what happens before and after the newsmaking events.

CHAPTER 1

HEALTH AND WELLNESS

Highlights of this chapter:

This chapter aims to put forth a fundamental concept about the overall health and well-being of teenagers in terms of basic concepts like diet, nutrition, and exercise. Main topics of discussion will be:

- *Healthy Weight, Nutritional Needs, and Healthy Diet*
- *Physical Activity and Exercise*
- *Water*
- *Unhealthy Eating Habits*
- *Fats*
- *Immune System*
- *Sleep*

HEALTHY DIET AND HEALTHY WEIGHT

For a healthy and disease-free existence, the intake of healthy nutrients is vital, particularly for teenagers due to extremely high-energy demands of their age group. You may have heard this before, but have you ever imagined what increases the nutritional requirements?

The body of an adolescent is a site of tremendous biochemical, physiological, and hormonal changes. At the time of puberty, the release of estrogen in females and testosterone in males increases significantly, producing effects such as:

- Growth spurts (rapid increase in height and development)
- Growth of muscles and body tissues
- A high basal metabolic rate (suggesting that you spend a lot of energy at rest), to list a few

Consuming a high quality diet that supplies great nutritional value in a "balanced manner" is highly recommended. Such a diet excludes junk foods (like snacks, burgers, and soda) that are low in nutritional value and usually considered bad for your health.

What are some healthy sources of a nutritious diet?

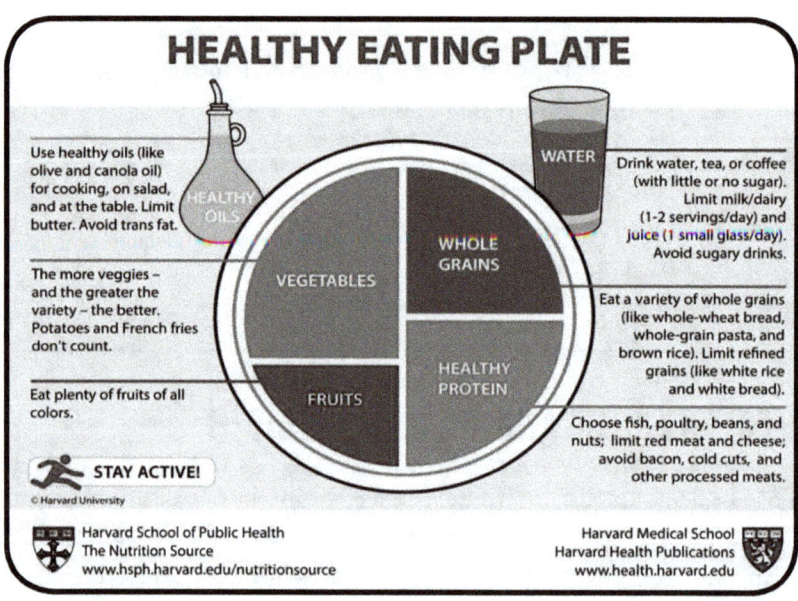

A balanced diet is comprised of a healthy intake of vegetables, fruits, healthy proteins, and whole grains. Foods that are rich in bad quality fats (like cholesterol or low-density lipoproteins) should be avoided, as they may lead to several health issues.

Here is the breakdown of the Healthy Eating Plate

- 50% of your food intake should be comprised of fruits and vegetables
- 25% of the plate should be made up of whole grains; such as quinoa, oats, wheat berries, whole wheat pasta, barley, and brown rice
- Remaining 25% should be supplied by healthy protein sources (fish, poultry, beans, and nuts). Avoid processed meat varieties.

Basic Principles of Healthy Nutrition:

Adolescents, as well as adults, who develop a habit of consuming high quality, nutrient dense foods tend to live a happier, healthier life. Currently, nutritionists and healthcare providers advise utilizing the Alternate Healthy Eating Index to assess and calculate your health and nutritional status.

The basic guidelines/ recommendations include:

1. Incorporation of eleven (11) components in the daily diet. This includes dairy products, fat, sodium, multi-vitamins, cholesterol, poultry/ fish, vegetables, bread/grains, meat, nuts and seeds, along with fruits.
2. Following a healthy diet over a period of 10 years or more can substantially reduce the risk of developing metabolic and medical conditions (discussed in detail in Chapter 4).
3. If you are consuming carbohydrates, it is more important to focus on the type of carbohydrate and not the percentage or amount of carbohydrate. For example, choosing whole grains, fruits and vegetables for carbohydrate consumption is far superior to French fries or bakery items. Obviously, in this scenario, the type of carb matters more than the amount or proportion of calories.

4. It is very important to maintain a healthy intake of high quality fats (or lipids). Lipids help in delivering fat-soluble vitamins and hormones across different parts of the body, in addition to assisting in the rejuvenation process of brain cells. Healthy sources include olive, canola, sunflower, soy and peanut oil.

A little about caloric intake and calorie distribution of foods:

It was traditionally believed that a large chunk of your caloric intake should be from carbohydrates, a fair percentage from proteins, and the intake of fat should ideally not exceed 5 – 15% of your total caloric intake. Is that a correct assessment or golden rule that can be applied to all individuals?

Review the following three scenarios below and consider if it is logical to provide the same type and proportions of food to all four.

Case 1:

Your 65-year-old grandpa, who is now retired, suffers from a few medical issues. His only physical activity is a 15 minute-walk before bedtime.

Case 2:

Your father, who works as a financial advisor at a local bank, has long and hectic work hours. But he still manages to take out some time for golfing and swimming.

Case 3:

Your younger sister, who has just turned 13, spends most of her time cycling and engaged in other outdoor activities.

Obviously, the amount of caloric intake depends entirely on an individual's age, height, gender, basal metabolic rate, amount of physical activity and other similar parameters. Taking a keen interest in maintaining a healthy nutritional intake is highly recommended, not just in terms of nutrients as suggested by HEALTHY EATING PLATE, but also in terms of calories.

Here is a reference range for optimal calorie intake according to age, gender and level of physical activity.

	MALES				FEMALES		
Activity level	Sedentary*	Mod. active*	Active*	Activity level	Sedentary*	Mod. active*	Active*
AGE				AGE			
2	1000	1000	1000	2	1000	1000	1000
3	1000	1400	1400	3	1000	1200	1400
4	1200	1400	1600	4	1200	1400	1400
5	1200	1400	1600	5	1200	1400	1600
6	1400	1600	1800	6	1200	1400	1600
7	1400	1600	1800	7	1200	1600	1800
8	1400	1600	2000	8	1400	1600	1800
9	1600	1800	2000	9	1400	1600	1800
10	1600	1800	2200	10	1400	1800	2000
11	1800	2000	2200	11	1600	1800	2000
12	1800	2200	2400	12	1600	2000	2200
13	2000	2200	2600	13	1600	2000	2200
14	2000	2400	2800	14	1800	2000	2400
15	2200	2600	3000	16	1800	2000	2400
16	2400	2800	3200	16	1800	2000	2400
17	2400	2800	3200	17	1800	2000	2400
18	2400	2800	3200	18	1800	2000	2400
19-20	2600	2800	3000	19-20	2000	2200	2400
21-25	2400	2600	3000	21-25	2000	2200	2400
26-30	2400	2600	3000	26-30	1800	2000	2400
31-35	2400	2600	3000	31-35	1800	2000	2200
36-40	2400	2600	2800	36-40	1800	2000	2200
41-45	2200	2600	2800	41-45	1800	2000	2200
46-50	2200	2400	2800	46-50	1800	2000	2200
51-55	2200	2400	2800	51-55	1600	1800	2200
56-60	2200	2400	2600	56-60	1600	1800	2200
61-65	2000	2400	2600	61-65	1600	1800	2000
66-70	2000	2200	2600	66-70	1600	1800	2000
71-75	2000	2200	2600	71-75	1600	1800	2000
76 and up	2004	2200	2400	76 and up	1600	1800	2000

Note: This chart is to be an estimate only. Calories needed may vary depending on a variety of other factors.

Vitamins and Minerals

Vitamins and minerals are classified under micronutrients that should be consumed in extremely small doses (like micrograms or even less) in order to speed up the process of metabolism and perform major biological activities. It is important to keep in mind that deficiency of such nutrients can lead to variety of health issues, but the full-blown symptoms of deficiencies may take some time to manifest.

Besides macronutrients, a growing teen also require healthy micronutrients in recommended amounts; such as:

- **Calcium** that is required for healthy bones and teeth. It can be obtained from green leafy vegetables, dried beans, fish, soybeans, tofu, and nuts.
- Citrus fruits (such as oranges and lemons), tomatoes, and potatoes are all good sources of **vitamin C**, which is essential for healthy skin and good for the immune system as well. Vitamin C is also essential for absorption of iron from our food.
- Fish oil (such as salmon and tuna), fortified (added nutrient) orange juice, mushrooms, and egg yolk are good sources of dietary **Vitamin D**, which helps in proper absorption of calcium that is required for healthy bones. Early morning sunlight is considered the best source of Vitamin D.
- Carrot, green vegetables, butter and apricots are good sources of **Vitamin A**, which is required for healthy skin and good vision.
- **Iron** is considered necessary to maintain healthy circulation by replacing dead and damaged red blood cells in the bloodstream and contributing to hematopoiesis (the formation of blood cells). It can be obtained from pulses, green vegetables, and fortified (added nutrients) cereals, fish, nuts, and meat.

- **Folic acid**, another nutrient essential for healthy blood, can be obtained from green vegetables and brown rice, as well as fortified bread and breakfast cereals.
- Fish is usually considered as the best source of protein, vitamins, and minerals. Teens should consume at least two servings of fish per week. Oily fish, such as salmon and tuna, also contain omega 3 fatty acids, which are good for health and a great source of energy too.

Eating Disorders:

There are several varieties of eating disorders. Healthcare providers, media managers, and politicians blame obesity (or overeating) for health issues; the fact is under-eating or poor dietary habits are equally to be blamed.

Are you aware that the prevalence of eating disorders is very high in the general population?

Here are a few noteworthy facts as to why you should pay attention to the text in this chapter.

- *50% of individuals who have eating disorders also develop moderate depression.*
- *Only 10% of individuals realize that they are suffering from an eating disorder and therefore require treatment*
- *86% of the eating disorders are reported in teenagers (under 20 years of age)*
- *If you are a male, the overall prevalence of eating disorders is 10-15%*
- *Approximately 50% of females and 33% of males admit to adopting abnormal eating habits to maintain their body weight (such as vomiting, purging, use of laxatives, dieting or even starving themselves).*

Do you think you are suffering from eating disorders too?

Here is a little test that is conventionally used in clinics to screen eating disorders amongst teens (be honest to yourself while taking the test).

Table 1 - DSM-IV-TR criteria for eating disorders associated with overweight and obesity

Bulimia Nervosa (types: purging, nonpurging)
- Recurrent episodes of binge eating
- Recurrent inappropriate compensatory behaviors to prevent weight gain
- Binge eating and inappropriate compensatory behavior occur at least twice a week far 3 months
- Self-evaluation unduly influenced by body shape and weight

Eating Disorder Nei Otherwise Specified

Disorder of eating that do not meet criteria for anorexia nervosa or bulimia nervosa.
- Female patient has regular menses
- Current weight is at least >85% expected
- Uses inappropriate compensatory behavior after eating small amounts of food
- Repeatedly chews and spits out large amounts of foods

   Binge Elating Disorder
   - Recurrent episodes of binge eating without vomiting or laxative obese
   - Often associated wish obesity
   - Currently listed in appendix of DSM-IV-TR

   Night Eating Syndrome
   - Morning anorexia
   - Increased appetite in the evening
   - Difficulty falling asleep
   - Patients can have amnesia for night eating

DSM-IV-TR, *Diagnostic and Statistical Manual of Mental Disorders, 4th Edition, Text Revision.*

How to maintain a healthy weight

Whatever you consume is utilized in different metabolic activities. If you eat a diet high in sugar (which is glucose and fructose), the excess sugar gets stored in the liver for later fuel or energy. If the liver's storage capacity is exceeded, the extra sugar turns into fat and is deposited in other tissues of the body (like the waist, face, buttocks, abdomen, love-handles and chest). If no intervention or modification in your diet is made, you will become obese (*learn more about obesity in Chapter 4*).

What should you know about maintaining a healthy weight?

A healthy weight is directly related to your diet. If you consume a healthy diet, you will have a healthy weight. A few tips that you should keep in mind for the maintenance of a healthy weight are:

- Intake of carbonated drinks (soda) and sugar-rich diet (sweets and cakes) should be eliminated, or at least cut down.
- Greatly decrease, or if possible eliminate, your intake of processed foods, such as burgers, chips and many other junk foods.
- Consume healthy food at intervals (starving is definitely bad for your body and your goal of maintaining a healthy weight).
- Make vegetables and fruits a part of your daily diet.
- It is generally recommended to eat less than 6g of salt per day. A higher intake of salt may lead to diseases like hypertension and cardiac dysfunction, but most importantly, the sodium in salt retains water in the body, causing bloating.
- Eat according to your weight and degree of metabolism/activity and most importantly, eat a variety of foods.

A lot of people today are adopting exclusive vegan diet as a method of maintaining a healthy weight. Is it actually helpful?
Let's discuss…

A balanced diet should contain sufficient quantities of fats, protein, and carbohydrates. The requirements for protein are even higher in growing adolescents. So if you are consuming a vegetarian or vegan diet, be sure you get enough protein from other sources like vegetables, beans, nuts, tofu, and lentils.

Healthcare providers advise continuing the Healthy Eating Plate regimen. You can replace proteins with healthy grains and other high-quality protein sources such as fish and eggs, (unless you are vegan), and pulses as an alternative to eating meat and/or fish.

UNHEALTHY EATING HABITS

First of all, it is important to understand that unhealthy eating habits do not always mean consumption of junk food. It has other dimensions as well; for example:

Excessive consumption of some otherwise healthy foods in unhealthy proportions can also cause harm. One good example is carbohydrates that are required for the generation of energy; yet if you consume too much of a particular type of carbohydrate or even fats (or any other micro- or macronutrient), the chances of nutritional hazards increase.

Some logical questions that may arise in this situation are:

- How do I know what nutrients to consume?
- How do I ensure a healthy intake of each nutrient?

And the answer to both the questions is the same…by educating yourself and learning more about the types of nutrients.

Difference between Sucrose, Glucose, and Fructose

These are commonly known as simple sugars and are listed as vital carbohydrates. Glucose, fructose, and sucrose provide the same quantity of energy, but their processing and usage in the body varies. Carbohydrates are categorized as monosaccharides, disaccharides, or polysaccharides. The basic and simple carbohydrate is monosaccharides, which are made with a single unit of sugar. Fructose and glucose are monosaccharides and further provide a base for building sucrose (a disaccharide). This shows that disaccharides are made from linked sugar molecule pairs or when two monosaccharides are joined together by discarding the water molecule.

Sucrose

Sucrose is attained from sugar beets or sugar cane and its common name is table sugar. It is naturally present in several vegetables and fruits. When a person consume sucrose, it decomposes into glucose and fructose sugar units by the enzyme namely beta fructosidase. Both the sugars are then performing their individual mechanism. The human body utilizes glucose to make its energy, whereas excess energy from fructose is stored for synthesizing fats, if not required currently by the body.

Facts about sucrose and excessive fructose intake:

Researchers and investigators have conducted a series of experiments on animal subjects to see the response to certain diets. In one of these experiments that were conducted to see how rats respond to high fructose and sucrose diets, it was reported that the weight gain observed was almost instant.

Is this even possible?

Indeed it is. You may have read about the process of osmosis (if you didn't, ask your biology teacher). In fact, it will be much more fun if you conduct a simple experiment at home.

Activity to see how carbohydrates (sugar) can lead to bloating

1. *Put some raisins in a bowl*
2. *Fill the bowl with water and let them sit for a few hours*

3. *Check the bowl and the raisins in a few hours*
4. *You will see the raisins are now plump (filled with water)*

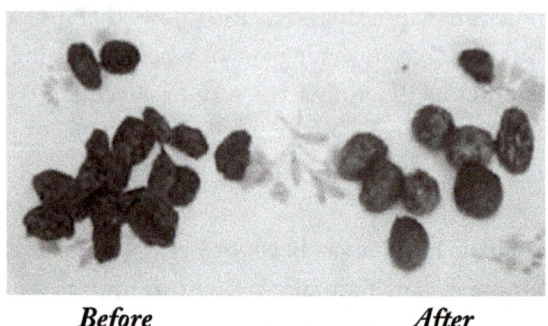

Before   **After**

The carbohydrates attract water, and a higher intake of carbs can eventually lead to a subsequent accumulation of water, leading to bloating and weight gain.

Here is what scientists observed when they fed fructose and sucrose rich diets to rats.

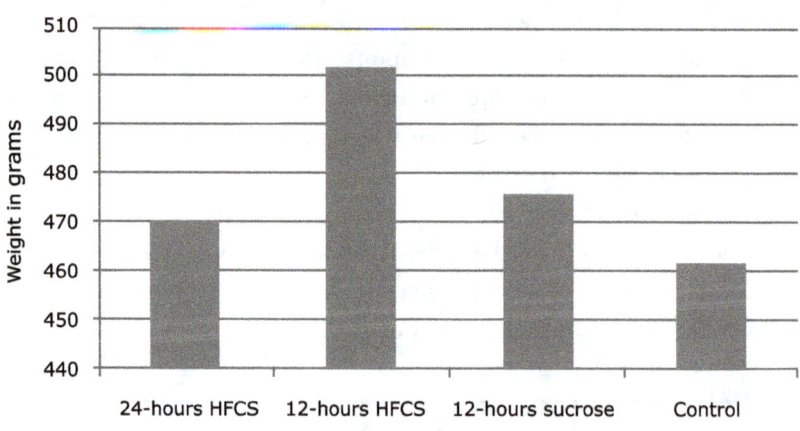

http://weightology.net/weightologyweekly/?page_id=19

Other hazardous effects of excessive sucrose and fructose intake are listed in the table below

Raise your blood pressure, and cause nocturnal hypertension	Insulin resistance/ Type 2 Diabetes	Non-alcoholic fatty liver disease (NAFLD)
Raise your uric acid levels, which can result in gout and/or metabolic syndrome	Accelerate the progression of chronic kidney disease	Intracranial atherosclerosis (narrowing and hardening of the arteries in your skull)
Exacerbate cardiac abnormalities if you're deficient in copper	Have a genotoxic effect on the colon	Promote metastasis in breast cancer patients
Cause tubulointerstitial injury (injury to the tubules and interstitial tissue of your kidney)	Promotes obesity and related health problems and diseases	Promotes pancreatic cancer growth

Glucose

It is one of the most important monosaccharides required by the human body to produce energy. It is also referred to as blood sugar because it flows in the blood. Glucose depends upon hexokinase and glucokinase enzymes for initiating metabolism process. The human body has the ability to process most of the carbohydrates to produce glucose, which is utilized immediately for energy production, can be stored in the cells of muscles, or can be stored in the liver as glycogen for use later when needed. When glucose levels rise in the blood, the hormone insulin is secreted by the pancreas to facilitate the admission of glucose into various cells.

Fructose

Fructose is a kind of sugar that is naturally available in several vegetables and fruits. It is included especially in several beverages like sodas to enhance the flavor of drinks. The working of fructose is entirely different as compared to other sugars due to its unique metabolic process.

Fructose does not provide energy to the brain and muscles; rather, it is metabolized only in the liver and depends on fructokinase to start its metabolic process.

This is one of the primary reasons why healthcare providers advise against consumption of excessive quantities of fructose. In addition:

- Fructose is fat producing or more lipogenic as compared to glucose.
- Unlike glucose, fructose does not release insulin and doesn't arouse leptin hormone (a hormone produced by fat cells that play a role in hunger and metabolism) production, which is responsible for regulating energy consumption and its expenditure.

Due to these factors, a diet with high fructose levels should be avoided as it behaves as fat in the body. Here are the effects of fructose in your body.

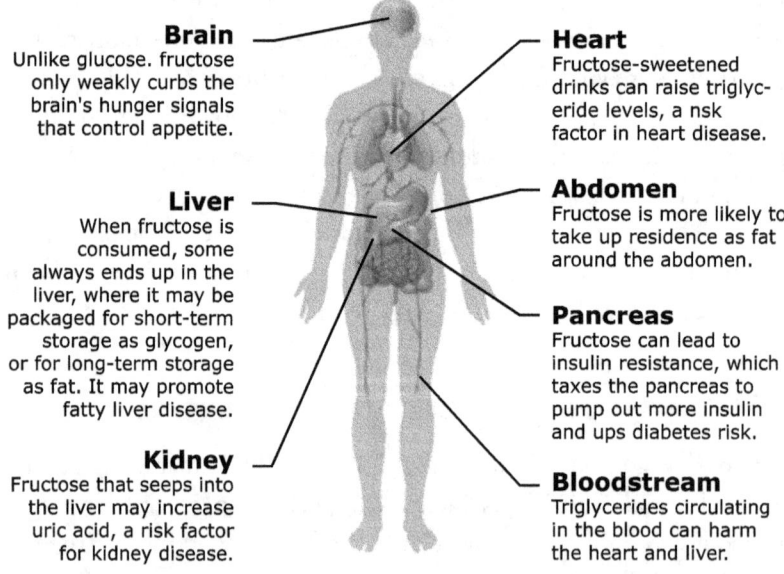

Brain
Unlike glucose, fructose only weakly curbs the brain's hunger signals that control appetite.

Heart
Fructose-sweetened drinks can raise triglyceride levels, a risk factor in heart disease.

Liver
When fructose is consumed, some always ends up in the liver, where it may be packaged for short-term storage as glycogen, or for long-term storage as fat. It may promote fatty liver disease.

Abdomen
Fructose is more likely to take up residence as fat around the abdomen.

Pancreas
Fructose can lead to insulin resistance, which taxes the pancreas to pump out more insulin and ups diabetes risk.

Kidney
Fructose that seeps into the liver may increase uric acid, a risk factor for kidney disease.

Bloodstream
Triglycerides circulating in the blood can harm the heart and liver.

https://www.sciencenews.org/article/sweet-confusion

The Truth About High Fructose Corn Syrup

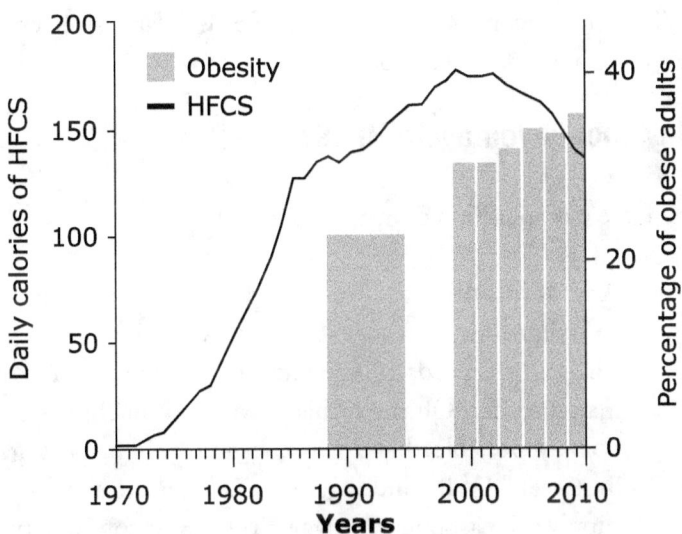

Are you aware that an average Westerner consumes 0 – 60 pounds of High Fructose Corn Syrup (HFCS) each year? In addition, high consumption of HFCS is directly implicated as an important factor in the pathogenesis of diabetes, insulin resistance, obesity, and cardiovascular issues.

High fructose corn syrup was introduced in the 1970s as a replacement sweetening agent to sucrose. Initially, it was believed that HFCS was a better option as compared to sucrose due to its ease of use and more functional and stable characteristics. However, in subsequent years, further research proved that HFCS is not only hazardous to your health, but is also a leading cause of several health issues as suggested by the research report published in the *American Journal of Clinical Nutrition*.

The chemical composition of fructose is different. Instead of 50:50 fructose and glucose combination, high fructose corn syrup is available in 55 molecules of fructose to 45 molecules of glucose, which hampers normal metabolism within the body after ingestion.

The most common sources of HFCS are sweetened beverages and processed foods.

Why should you avoid HFCS?

There are a myriad of reasons; for example:

- Any form of sugar is hazardous, but the risk of complications increases if the intake of high fructose corn syrup exceeds 140 pounds per person per year. You may assume, "Oh man, this is way too much; there is no way possible that I can consume this much sugar in a year." Well think again. A 20-ounce can of soda supply 17 teaspoons of sugar. Even if you consume two cans of soda per day; you can easily cross this limit of HFCS intake (don't forget other sources of sugar that you consume).
- As expected, when you consume a bolus of fructose, the sugar directly gains access into the bloodstream (due to different digestive mechanism) and promotes lipogenesis in the liver that further leads to liver dysfunction.
- There is always a very high risk of mercury contamination with an intake of high fructose corn syrup. In the diet of an average America, high fructose corn syrup comprises about 20% of the diet.
- Due to the composition, chemistry, and nature of HFCS, it is usually present in foods that are relatively unhealthy and low in nutrient quality. If your intake of HFCS foods is high, it clearly indicates that your overall quality of food intake is poor.

Report by GA Berry suggested:

"Most conservative estimate of the consumption of HFCS indicates a daily average of 132 kcal for all Americans aged ≥ 2 y, and the top 20% of consumers of caloric sweeteners ingest 316 kcal from HFCS/d. The increased use of HFCS in the United States mirrors the rapid increase in obesity".

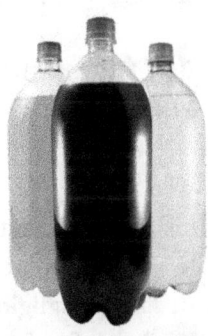

High Fructose Corn Syrup is in EVERYTHING!

Its been linked and blame for obesity, diabetes and now...

HIGH BLOOD PRESSURE!

Some sources of high fructose corn syrup are:
Bread, whipped cream, crackers, tomato-based sauces, snacks, yogurt, breakfast pastries, sodas, fruit drinks, cereals, ice creams, drink mixes, candy, jams, jellies, and cereals.

HEALTHY AND UNHEALTHY FATS

Before we discuss nutrition in much greater detail, let's test your knowledge of fats.

Answer **true or false** to the following questions:

1. *Teens should avoid lipids / fats in order to maintain their body weight*
2. *All fatty sources are bad for health.*

3. *High intake of all fats increases the risk of cardiac diseases and cholesterol metabolism issues*
4. *High intake of fat causes obesity*

I am hoping your answer to all the questions listed above is NO. If you picked 'Yes' for any of the questions listed above; you must read the text below.

Let's review these questions one by one.

Teens should avoid lipids / fats in order to maintain their body weight

Absolutely not…Teens require healthy fats more than adults for growth and development. This is because fats serve as a medium or channel to transport hormones and fat soluble vitamins in the body. If you decrease your intake of fat to negligible levels, the risk of fat soluble vitamins and hormone deficiency increases several folds that will ultimately affect growth and development.

All fatty sources are bad for health

Once again, not all dietary sources of lipids are bad for health. Besides transporting hormones and vitamins, fat is also a reserved form of energy that keeps your body warm and energized when you exercise or during periods when your intake is low due to fasting, illness, or while exercising.

Eat real fat to:

- Promote fat burning
- Build muscle faster
- Curb cravings for junk food
- Supply your body with essential nutrients
- Better absorb vitamins and antioxidants

High intake of all fats increases your risk of cardiac diseases and cholesterol metabolism issues

Did you know that fats are actually protective against heart diseases?

Good quality lipids (like high-density lipoproteins) are cardio-protective as these are high in Vitamin E and antioxidants to ward off free radicals and disease causing agents.

High intake of fat causes obesity

Once again, intake of high-quality fats increases the basal metabolic rate, which helps in losing weight instead of gaining it.

There are many sources of obtaining dietary fat, but it is highly advised to consume more of the good fat foods rather than food with zero fats. If you have a high tendency to develop cardiac issues (due to strong family history of heart diseases or inherited/ genetic conditions that predispose you to cardiac illness), do not avoid fat. Instead, replace trans fats with good fats and limit saturated fats intake by deducting full fat dairy products and red meat. Add fish, beans, and nuts, and/ or poultry, red meat, and whole milk (in moderation) to your diet. Consume omega 3 fats daily from walnuts, fish, flaxseed oil, soybean oil, or canola oil.

It is important to limit your fat intake, according to the recommendations of USDA that is:

- Limit your total fat intake to up to 35% of calories.
- Consume less than 10% of saturated fats in your daily calories
- Consume 1% of trans fats in your daily calories.

Eliminate trans fat from your daily diet

When considering healthy fats, it is essential to eliminate the consumption of trans fats. According to the conclusion of several studies, trans fats are not healthy for the human body. They can cause several serious health problems, ranging with heart diseases to cancer. When talking about trans fats, a picture of margarine flashed in our minds. Margarines are overloaded with trans fats. In a Western diet, trans fats are primarily obtained from snack foods and baked goods, which are prepared commercially. The following are some examples of trans fats sources (which are not good for you):

- Baked goods such as crackers, cookies, muffins, cakes, pizza dough, pie crusts, etc.
- Fried foods such as French fries, doughnuts, chicken nuggets, fried chicken, etc.
- Snack foods such as potato chips, tortilla chips, corn chips, microwave or packaged popcorn, candy, etc.
- Solid fats such as semi-solid vegetable shortening and stick margarine
- Pre-mixed products such as chocolate drink mix, cake mix, and pancake mix.

Limit and reduce saturated fats consumption

The following tips will be helpful in limiting your consumption of saturated fats:

- Eat chicken and fish more and cut red meat from your diet.
- Stick with white meat, as it has a minimum of saturated fats, and approach for lean cut meat.
- Avoid frying meat; instead, broil, grill, or bake it.
- Remove chicken's skin before eating and trim fat off before cooking it.
- Avoid deep fried items and breaded meats.
- Use canola oil or olive oil instead of using butter or lard.
- Do not consume cheese sauces and creams.

Add good fats in diet

To obtain good mono and polyunsaturated fats, consume nuts, fish, seeds, and vegetable oils.

- Cook your food with olive oil
- Consume more avocados
- Add nuts in you dishes
- Prepare the salad dressing yourself and avoid commercially available dressings.

WATER

Most of you have a lot of concerns about eating healthy; but how many of you have actually tried looking for information about water?

You must be wondering, "What is there about water to search?"

Well, actually a lot. Do you know how much water you should consume every day?

- 8 glasses?
- 2 liters?
- 12 cups?

All the answers are wrong. You will figure out the correct answer by the end of this chapter.

Water is an excellent solvent that filters your blood, and removes all the impurities, toxins, chemicals, breakdown products, and drugs from your body. The importance of water is so great that:

- You cannot survive without water for three days (whereas, you can survive without any food for four to six weeks)
- Low water intake can lead to diseases, infections, and end-organ damage.

What are the benefits of water?

What Does Water do for You?

Forms saliva (digestion)

Keeps mucousal membranes moist

Allows body's cells to grow, reproduce and survive

Flushes body waste, mainly in urine

Lubricates joints

Water is the major component of most body parts

Needed by the brain to manufacture hormones and neurotransmitters

Regulates body temperature (sweating and respiration)

Acts as a shock absorber for brain and spinal cord

Converts food to components needed for survival - digestion

Helps deliver oxygen all over the body

Besides the few basic listed benefits, there are numerous other benefits of water:

1. Water improves the integrity of membranes that helps in decreasing the risk of dehydration associated disorders.
2. Water improves the flow of nerve impulses. If you get dehydrated, your mental performance and physical functional capacity decreases.
3. Water intake helps in the regulation of body temperature. When you pass urine or perspire, the body loses some of the unnecessary heat too.
4. Ample water intake is helpful in minimizing the risk of skin diseases and infections like eczema, arthritis, acne, etc.
5. Blood is comprised of 80 – 85% water. The water or fluid part helps in maintaining blood pressure.

6. Adequate water intake is needed for strong joints, muscle function, and productive cartilage.
7. Water assists in maintaining normal digestive processes and reduces the risk of constipation and gut allergies/inflammatory disorders.

How much water do you really need per day?

Having read all the benefits of water ; have you changed the answer?

Here is what you should see:

Minimum Daily Requirement for Water	
Population Group	**Minimum Daily Requirements**
Infants	
Birth to less than 6 months	800 ml
6 to 12 months	1000 ml
Children (1-18 y)	
Wt (kg)	
10-20	1000 ml + 50ml/kg for each excess kg
>20	1500 ml + 20 ml/kg for each excess kg
Adults 18+	2500 ml
Older persons, 65 and above	1500 ml
Pregnant women	Additional 300 ml
Lactation Women, 1st 6 months	Additional 750 to 1000 ml

So although an average teen or adult should drink at least 2.5 liters of water per day, is it absolute?

Definitely a big NO

- If you work out or exercise daily; you need more water

- If you live in hot climatic conditions; you need more water

Periods of illness, recovery period, and intake of highly processed or high salt foods are some other conditions that increase your recommended intake of water. It is therefore recommended by healthcare providers to maintain steady water intake (only by following your thirst). Do not force yourself to drink water just to curb your appetite or hunger. Drink water to promote health and well-being.

*A good rule of thumb is to drink half your body weight in ounces.
For example: If you weigh 120 pounds, you should drink at least 60 ounces of water per day.

Some healthy tips to improve your water intake:

- Avoid caffeinated beverages, alcohol, and a high salt diet that causes relative dehydration.
- Add lemon or natural flavor in water if you don't like plain water.
- Drink cold water (if you exercise vigorously, or want to burn a few extra calories)
- Drink warm water (for better hydration, digestion, and detoxification)

PHYSICAL ACTIVITY AND EXERCISE

Most teens today (almost all over the world) have become less active and spend most of their day watching television, in front of a computer on the Internet, texting or calling their friends, and on social media. According to a recent survey, adolescents and teens spend most of their time on social media forums or engaged in other forms of sedentary activities, like video games, movies, music, studies, etc.

What are some helpful tips that can make you more dynamic?

A few tips that can help in increasing your physical activity rate are:

- Choose interactive sports (and be friends with physically as well as socially active individuals)
- Join your school sports teams
- Be a part of camping trips with your school mates/classmates
- Host gatherings outdoors instead of indoors
- Get a bicycle or skateboard (and you will find tons of other adolescents your age in nearby parks)
- Slowly incorporate activities and try to involve your friends or siblings in the activities (to make it more fun)
- Join aerobics, dance classes, yoga or similar training sessions instead of employing conventional gym exercises.

Healthcare providers suggest that teenagers who adopt regular exercise and physical activity in their daily routine are more productive, healthy, and energetic.

If you don't have a lot of time, do not engage yourself in long workout sessions. It is more important to be consistent and regular rather than performing vigorous physical activity once in a while.

Time needed depends on effort

Light Effort 60 minutes	Moderate Effort 30-60 minutes	Vigorous Effort 20-30 minutes
• Light walking • Volleyball • Easy gardening • Stretching	• Brisk walking • Biking • Raking leaves • Swimming • Dancing • Water aerobics	• Aerobics • Jogging • Hockey • Basketball • Fast swimming • Fast dancing

How does it feel?
How warm am I? What is my breathing like?

• Starting to feel warm • Slight increase in breathing rate	• Warmer • Greater increase in breathing rate	• Quite warm • More out of breath

Range needed to stay healthy

What are the benefits of Physical activity/exercise?

Exercise or physical activity is helpful in promoting a number of benefits.

Physical benefits:

Regular physical activity is helpful in:

- Building of muscles
- Remodeling of bones
- Conditioning of connective tissue framework

Medical Benefits:

- Promote healthy metabolism
- Helps in regulating normal healthy weight
- Regulate serum glucose levels
- Regulate the secretion of insulin
- Reduce the risk of cardiac illnesses
- Minimize the risk of developing obesity, diabetes, and osteoporosis
- Reduce the risk of arthritis, joint diseases, and injuries

Psychological Benefits:

- Promotes delivery of oxygen rich blood to the brain
- Helps in the synthesis of hormones and chemical mediators that are required to maintain and uplift mood

How much exercise is good or acceptable?

While there are many adolescents who are not interested in physical activities or exercises at all, you will find many who spend most of their time in the gym or fitness center in order to build muscle mass or to lose weight (or as a result of other hidden psychological factors, such as body dysmorphic syndrome in which adolescents always feel they are ugly or less attractive).

Over-exercising is a common teen obsession that may lead to harmful complications in some cases. In his research article published in *International Journal of Mental Health and Addiction* Attila Szabo reported that the prevalence of exercise addiction in the adolescent population is 3.6 to 6.9%. Just like any medicine, exercising has its benefits. It helps in maintaining overall physical and mental health, helps in strengthening the bones and muscles, and allows us to get rid of extra unwanted body weight.

Healthcare providers advise regular physical activity and exercise to achieve numerous health benefits, but how many of us actually know:

- *How much exercise is desirable?*
- *If excessive exercise is even better for the body?*
- *Most importantly, if excessive physical activity can lead to any adverse effects?*

What happens when you over-exercise?

There are several reasons why we should limit our physical activity to recommended limits. Here are a few drawbacks of excessive exercising.

1. Muscle fatigue

Exercising directly involves the muscles and skeletal tissue elements. When a person exercises, the muscles stretch and contract, which increases the production of proteins. The resultant effect is muscle hypertrophy and increase in bulk, strength, and power.

On the contrary, over-exercising creates a state of overloading that makes it difficult for muscles to function properly. Here's how:

- Exercising muscles require energy in the form of substrate (like glucose or glycogen). Excessive exercise can lead to depletion of energy stores
- As a result of activity, the exercising muscles produce waste products (like lactic acid) as a breakdown product of metabolism. When the rate of lactic acid production exceeds the rate of excretion, muscles develop soreness and pain.

2. Increased risk of musculoskeletal injuries:

Over-exercising also increases the risk of injuries that may be minor in the beginning, but with over-exercising, it becomes even more difficult to heal the injuries. In poorly managed cases, the risk of conditions like Delayed Onset Muscle Soreness (DOMS), arthritis, stress fractures, and other similar lesions increases considerably.

3. Chemical Reactions in tissues:

Healthcare providers and exercise physiologists believe that over-exercising can cause an alteration in stamina, increase the risk of injuries, and interfere with normal tissue regeneration or healing. The primary reason is the disruption of the body's normal chemical balance that directly interferes with immunity.

4. Death in extreme and poorly managed cases:

Life threatening conditions such as Rhabdomyolysis may occur. This condition is characterized by severe muscle wasting, which leads to the release and accumulation of the protein myoglobin. This causes kidney damage, resulting in decreased urine production and loss of electrolyte balance, causing the urgent need of dialysis. If this condition is not recognized in time, it may ultimately lead to death.

Other adverse effects of over-exercising on the body are:

- Contrary to popular belief, over-exercising can actually damage health instead of causing any good. Strenuous and unnecessary activity can deplete the body's muscles of oxygen and may lead to breathing problems. Gradually, the tolerance towards activity decreases, which also leads to persistent fatigue and a feeling of tiredness.
- An unhealthy exercise regimen also takes a toll on daily activities (persistent fatigue leads to moodiness, low energy levels, and overall low productivity)
- Over-exercise damages the musculoskeletal elements and thereby increases the risk of chronic inflammation, overuse

injury, arthritis, stress fractures, and eventually can require surgical intervention for correction.
- Exercising can cause dehydration and loss of electrolyte balance very quickly. These can be identified by persistent muscle cramping, nausea, vomiting and heart palpitations. Therefore, it is of utmost importance to avoid over-exercising and more importantly, keeping yourself hydrated at all times is vital.

SYMPTOMS OF OVERTRAINING SYNDROME		
Performance Issues	*Physiological Symptoms*	*Psychological Symptoms*
• Early Fatigue • Increased Heart Rate w/less Effort • Decreased Strength, Endurance, Speed and Coordination • Decreased Aerobic Capacity • Delayed Recovery	• Persistent Fatigue • On-going Muscle Soreness • Loss of Appetite • Excessive weight Loss • Excessive Loss of Body Fat • Irregular Menses • Increased Resting Heart Rate • Chronic Muscle Soreness • Increase in Overuse Injuries • Difficulty Sleeping • Frequent Colds or Infections	• Irritation or Anger • Depression • Difficulty in Concentration • Increased Sensitivity to Emotional Stress • Loss of Competitive Drive • Loss of Enthusiasm

http://mediconweb.com/exercise-and-fitness/signs-symptoms-effects-exercise-addiction-overtraining-syndrome/#.U0rKFvldX_I

When we exercise, we use carbohydrates as a fuel, which is the first source of our energy. Next comes the fat, which is what exercising should ideally target. However, over-exercising causes our body to turn to other sources, which include our muscles, leading to drastic side effects, such as increased weight loss and muscle damage.

What are some helpful strategies to prevent over-exercising?

If you are looking for a fast remedy to counter-balance or neutralize the effects of over-exercising, you may want to follow these tips:

- Instead of prolonging your exercise sessions, it is a far better idea to use more vigorous exercises to train your muscles and body.
- Increase your water intake to ensure excretion of toxic metabolic and chemical waste products from your body.
- Get ample rest (both physical and mental) after every exercise session to restore your chemical equilibrium

What are some factors that may lead to over-exercising?

Do you often find yourself obsessed with exercising? Some individuals have an addiction tendency towards exercising. Several factors, including feeling good about you, trying to overcome a negative body image phobia, etc., may contribute. Exercise causes the release of endorphins; these chemicals can cause euphoria and reduced stress levels. Therefore it is necessary to evaluate our reasons to exercise, along with the frequency with which we exercise.

Clive Long, in his research study published in *Behavioural and Cognitive Psychotherapy*, reported that over-exercising is a serious problem, but is often neglected. The author suggested that issues like over-exercising or exercise addiction often co-exist with eating disorders (especially anorexia nervosa).

Other commonly reported factors that often co-exist with over-exercising are:

- High levels of stress (due to personal, professional, or social reasons)
- Anxiety or depression
- Low self-esteem
- Negative body image (that also increases the risk of eating disorders and also promote other unhealthy activities).

It is recommended to identify secondary causes and factors that lead to over-exercising in order to devise a functional strategy to control these issues. For example, Long suggested that proper motivation, counseling, and behavioral therapy is effective in most of the cases.

Caroline Davis suggested that most cases of exercise addiction are associated with anorexia nervosa and starvation that further aggravates the damage to vital organs.

Expert and exercise trainers advise workout sessions of at least 90 minutes three times a week in order to decrease the risk of over-exercising and health hazards that follow.

What are the signs of over-exercising?

You may be overdoing it if you are:

- Feeling exhausted
- Sleeping more or less
- Feeling your legs are heavy
- Sore for days
- Losing motivation
- Unhappy or more moody

You can evaluate for yourself if you over-exercise or not, by answering these simple questions:

- Do you suffer extreme fatigue and tiredness all the time?
- Are you experiencing moderate weight loss without any changes in appetite?
- Do you often experience muscle or connective tissue injuries?
- If you miss an exercise session in a day, do you feel guilty about it?
- Are you experiencing changes in the sleep rhythm or appetite?
- Are you experiencing muscle weakness and heart palpitations?

If the answer to most of the questions above is YES, you may have to modify your exercise regimen.

One might imagine athletes to be spared from the adverse effects of over-exercising, but the sad truth is that no one is!

Over-exercising caused Rhabdomyolysis led to seven swimmers from South Carolina to have an ER visit in 2008, while in 2011, thirteen Iowa football players were hospitalized. This is because their bodies were constantly subjected to stress and overworking, causing them to weaken and lose their strength.

Stressful exercising regimens, when continued for long times, will ultimately lead to a strong dislike towards exercising altogether. Going through the same pain and side effects of over-exercising every single day will lead to a negative attitude in our lives and cause an exercising phobia in the end. Therefore, it is necessary to follow a regimen, as directed by an expert trainer, to gain maximum benefits and avoid any possible harmful effects.

So isn't it pretty confusing? Exercise is essential, yet if done more than recommended, exercise can harm your body and affects your health negatively. So what can be a possible solution?

Here is a set of recommended physical activities as advised by the healthcare providers for teenagers especially.

What are some exercises/physical activity tips that may prove effective and helpful for your health?

Healthy exercise should be engaging and fun, and for that it must have a range of variety, just in case you get bored and exhausted. Certainly healthy exercise doesn't revolve around elliptical machines, track running, or gyms. However, it certainly requires your cooperation by getting up on your feet in order to work out. Listed below is some anecdotal advice that you may use in your situation while doing a healthy work out.

At a slow pace try moving around a lot

Moving at a slow pace specifically refers to exercise that would keep your heart rate under 80% maximum. If you do something and find it difficult to breathe because you are hyperventilating, then this is not a slow pace at all.

Walking at a brisk pace is also counted as a slow pace, whereas jogging isn't. According to Thomas Jefferson, the best exercise is walking. A simple plain walk is free from all sorts of risk and is very beneficial.

For some more reduced cardio level exercises, go with hiking, which here means walking in a natural setting. You may also ride a bike, or even decide to go rowing or canoeing. A job where you have to be mostly on your feet will do too. In winter, you may go snowshoeing or skiing. You may even swim, indoors of course, or in a heated pool.

Avoid chronic cardio

Sometimes while racing for six hours or so, one may end up breaking this law, but it is okay to do so once in a blue moon. However, if you make it your habit, it will consequently lead to more risks of burning out the thyroid and adrenal glands, which in turn contribute to aging. Some people are genetically equipped to exercise more than 80% of the threshold and somehow do not end up causing any damage to them.

Jogging moderately or riding a bike for two to three hours is a piece of cake for some teens as if walking in the park. Do not beat yourself up because you are not in this category or are not so well genetically equipped. Follow the fundamental laws of fitness and you will do just fine.

Lifting heavy things

You may use free-weight objects for lifting, such as dumbbells, tires, trees and rocks. Simple body-weight exercises are even better, like lunges, squats, dips, pull-ups and push-ups. These exercises help in developing functional strength and assist in stimulation of natural body skills and movements. You may get nice toned muscles if you practice the routine on a regular basis. A bush workout will also be your key to fitness. It involves practicing leaping, climbing trees, and lifting rocks.

Sprint once in a while

Sprinting comes in with a lot of options. Athletes are already familiar with intervals. Sprinting is easiest for runners. Try doing sprints from 100-400 meters, but do not ignore coping with your breathing of course. Cyclists need to sprint for max efforts for a minute or two in a steep hill with a crest. For swimmers, sprinting a lap or two followed by recovery and more intervals is sufficient. Sprinting once a week is just fine, but you may do it 3-5 times a week.

Activity

1. *Analyse your physical activity regimen and compare it with the recommendations listed in the text.*
2. *Prepare a more functional physical activity regimen and maintain a journal to track your progress.*

IMMUNE SYSTEM

The defense mechanism of the body, which is responsible for detecting and fighting pathogens and promoting health and wellness, is the immune system. But what else should you know about the immune system?

Basically, we are exposed to hundreds of pathogens around us. You don't believe it? Let's review:

Cigarette smoking is believed to cause a variety of cancers (like esophageal, lung, stomach, colon, etc). You will learn more about it in subsequent chapters. Yet, despite being exposed to cigarette smoke (and other types of smoke), we don't develop cancer readily.

Likewise, we have hundreds of viruses and bacteria around us that try to attack and invade our body. Yet, with every exposure, we don't develop sickness or illness.

Why is that so?

This is because the human body is designed in a highly complicated yet functional manner.

Primary defense mechanisms of the body:

Dietary intake is one of the most convenient sources of bacterial or fungal invasion (not to forget the worms). Fortunately, we have a lot of protective mechanisms from the mouth to the anus that detect and kill those invaders. For example, stomach cells secrete a highly acidic solution (hydrochloric acid) that kills bacteria and other microorganisms to prevent diseases or illness.

- Any bacteria, virus, or fungi that evades the gut or gains access via the respiratory passageways is ultimately detected by defense cells—neutrophils, lymphocytes, monocytes, and macrophages—that engulf and destroy foreign invaders.
- Besides killing and destroying foreign invaders, the human body also prepares memory cells that store the identity of the foreign invaders so that if the same bacterial species invade our bodies again, the military of our body is more readily available with necessary ammunition to fight it.

What are 10 classic tips to boost your inherent immunity?

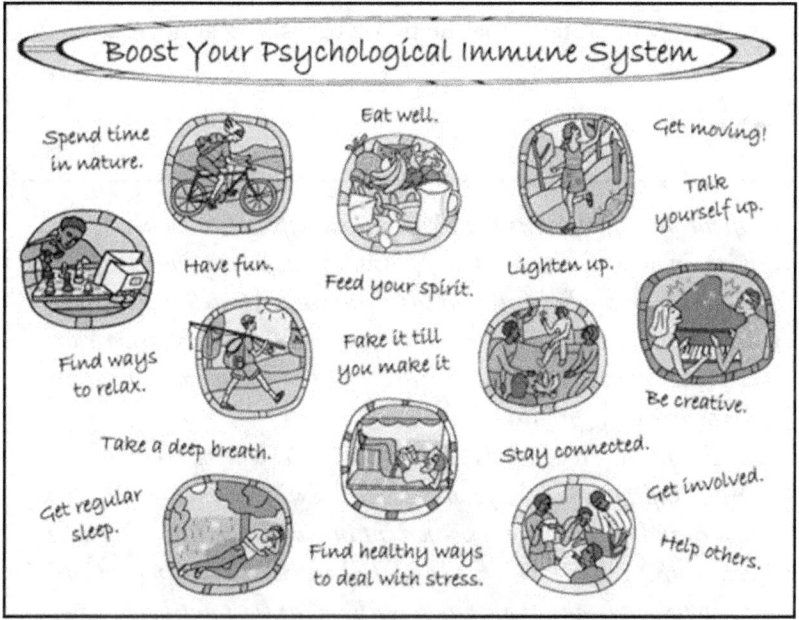

http://www.healingfromdepression.com/treating-depression-holistically.htm

Your body is designed by Nature to protect you from diseases, yet the basic condition is, "your body should be fit and strong." Here are a few tips to maintain the strength and stability of your body:

- Get ample sleep
- Eat healthy food
- Increase your intake of antioxidants
- Reduce stress
- Promote healthy living
- Eliminate toxins from your diet and life
- Be happy and love others (it acts as a tonic)
- Perform daily physical activity
- Meditate and perform yoga

- Perform stress relieving activities
- Avoid alcohol, carbonated beverages, high sugar intake and preservatives/ chemicals in your food
- Eat lean proteins that help in synthesizing antibodies

SLEEP

Oftentimes, adolescents are given the example of teens like Carey. Born in a middle-class family, Carey has always been a very responsible and obedient child. As a student, she excelled, but unlike most nerds, she is equally good in sports and other extracurricular activities. Fortunately, when she turned 15, she was also selected in the cheerleading group.

For just a 16-year-old high school student, it has now become fairly difficult to manage her studies, extracurricular activities, family and friends, and involvement in sports activities all at once. Her mother is quite concerned and she has tried explaining to Carey a few times already to give up something (at least until her exams) but Carey has something else in mind.

She was told by a friend that caffeine pills and energy drinks are fairly effective at increasing energy levels. In fact, she is quite happy with the results so far. Now she can stay up late at night (still active and productive) and of course manage her curricular and extracurricular activities

- Is there anything wrong in this picture perfect life of Carey?
- Are you juggling to maintain your curricular and extracurricular activities as well?
- How do you manage your time and maintain your productivity?

How Much Sleep Do You Really Need?	
Age	**Sleep Needs**
Newborns (0-2 months)	12-18 hours
Infants (3 to 11 months)	14 to 15 hours
Toddlers (1-3 years)	12 to 14 hours
Preschoolers (3-5 years)	11 to 13 hours
School-age children (5-10 years)	10 to 11 hours
Teens (10-17)	8.5-9.25 hours
Adults	7-9 hours

Source: *National Sleep Foundation*

The latest statistics suggested that the use of caffeine pills and energy drinks is increasing at an alarming rate among teens. For most adolescents, it is an easy shortcut to remain productive for long hours. According to the data recorded by the National Sleep Foundation:

- Only 20% of teens get the recommended amount of sleep (9 hours)
- More than 28% of adolescents doze off during active class sessions (prevalence of absent mindedness and low productivity is even greater, but unfortunately cannot be measured)

Quiz to assess if you are getting ample sleep or not?

- *How much sleep do you need each night?*
- *How many hours do you sleep each night?*
- *What is your daily caffeine intake? (Include tea, coffee, caffeinated beverages, coke and energy drinks*

(Review your answers from the text)

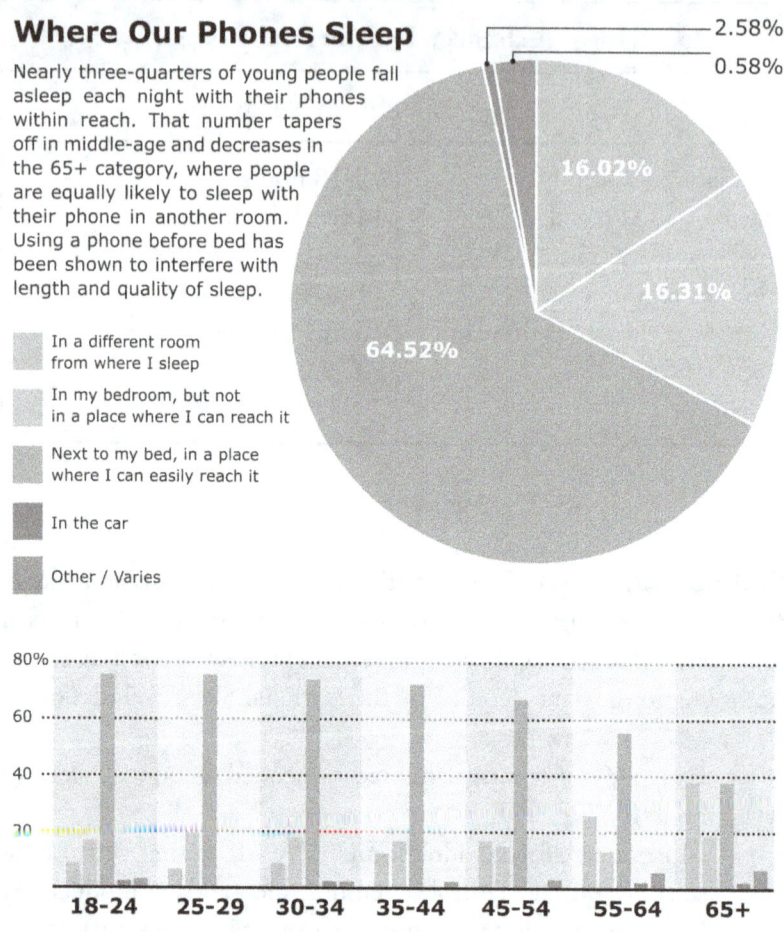

http://www.huffingtonpost.com/2013/02/15/phones-sleep-mobile-_n_2680805.html

Besides study and social activities, another cause of low sleep in teens is cellular phones and social media networks. Most teens like sleeping with their phones on or next to their bed so that they can stay up to chat with their friends' communication networks and similar activities.

What happens if you sleep too little?

Not being able to sleep one night due to an important exam, a sleepover, or a party is different than chronic abnormal sleeping habits. You should know that inadequate sleep can lead to:

- Depression, mood swings, and psychological disorders
- Poor capacity to deal with physical stressors and high risk of anxiety attacks, panic disorder, and even suicide
- Obesity
- High risk of heart diseases
- Sleepiness (only getting 6 hours of sleep or less can mimic intoxication)
- Poor performance at school and overall low energy levels that also decreases productivity
- Difficulty in performing simple tasks which are otherwise not difficult.

FEELING THE EFFECTS OF SLEEP DEPRIVATION

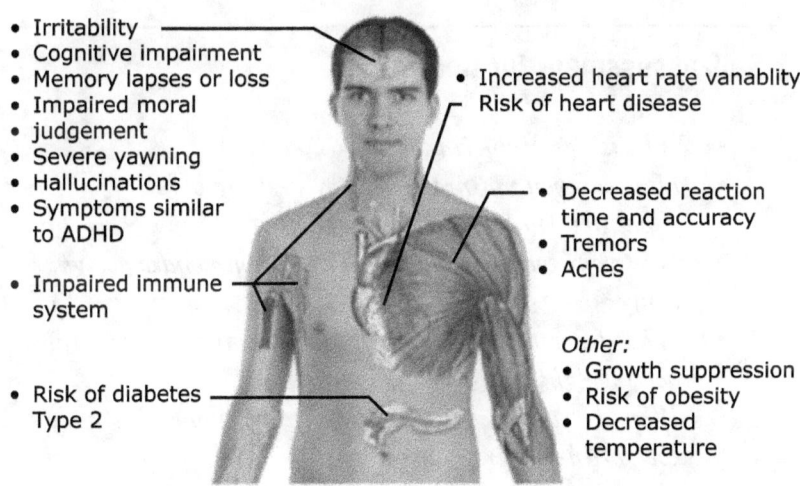

http://www.yourhealthdetective.com/2013/11/index.html

There is a high risk of deaths due to accidents while driving or performing complicated tasks when sleep deprived (data indicates that 37% teens fall asleep while driving).

How to maintain healthy sleeping habits?

- Perform daily physical activity (as mentioned previously, exercise causes muscle exhaustion and improves the quality of sleep)
- Eliminate or greatly decrease your intake of caffeinated beverages, especially after 4 PM
- Sips of water after dinner to avoid having to go to the bathroom during sleep
- Turn off your computer, television, and phone at least 1 hour before sleeping
- Avoid eating food or high sugar desserts before bedtime
- Keep your bedroom dark and noise-free
- Sleep at a particular time every night
- If you snore, or are extremely restless or tired during the day, having a (PSG) Polysomnogram can help guide treatment to help you achieve your "A" game.

Self-assessment for Chapter 1

- *Why is sleep important?*
- *How can you maintain healthy sleeping habits?*
- *What are you lacking in your diet?*
- *Does your weight fall within the recommended weight range?*
- *What interventions can you take to manage your ideal body weight?*
- *Why do you need you maintain recommended body weight in the first place?*
- *What happens when you over-exercise?*
- *How can you measure your exercise intensity?*
- *How much water should you drink on an average day? What are some factors that may increase your water intake?*

CHAPTER 2
PHYSICAL HEALTH

The aim of this chapter is to discuss some factors that may help in monitoring your overall health (in accordance with all the factors that we have discussed in Chapter 1).

Highlights of this chapter

- *Annual Physical*
- *Dental Health*
- *Eye Health*

ANNUAL PHYSICAL EXAMINATIONS

An annual checkup involves investigations about your health by a personal physician or a health care professional. This checkup is conducted yearly and should be made a priority not only for an individual, but for the whole family.

What does an annual checkup consist of?

Annual checkups (physical) consist of an examination of the following:

- Organs of the abdominal region
- Heart and lung function
- Spine alignment
- Neurological function

- Height
- Weight
- Oral hygiene
- ENT (ear, nose, and throat) evaluation

Who should get an annual physical examination?

- Teens with a history of metabolic or medical issues, such as heart conditions, chronic diseases like juvenile diabetes, or people with genetic tendencies to develop a disease should see a physician at intervals.
- Every individual above the age of 13 years should see a healthcare provider.
- Teens who have a history of mental illness, recognized psychological condition, obsession, or eating disorders should see a healthcare provider at intervals (and somewhat more frequently to see the response to therapy and if their overall health is satisfactory).

Why get an annual checkup?

- Primarily to prevent, identify, and treat any disease occurring at an early stage. This can prove very helpful in treatment.
- Teenagers especially need constant guidance and education about their personal hygiene. Any psychological or clinical diseases can be addressed at an early stage.
- To learn more about tips to maintain mental, physical, and sexual heath.

In the long run, prevention is better than cure.

EYE HEALTH

The eye is the exclusive visual sense of all our senses. Any disease to this organ can cause direct impairment of our visual senses. Some kinds of eye diseases remain without symptoms for a long time, therefore a periodic eye exam is of utmost importance.

Conditions such as iritis, conjunctivitis, cataract, or glaucoma are the most commonly occurring diseases that can be prevented or caught at an early stage with regular checkups. Also, people suffering from diseases that tend to harm other body organs over time such as diabetes and oligoarthritis (an inflammatory form of arthritis occasionally seen in youth) can affect our eyesight without symptoms occurring for a long time.

Unfortunately, a lot of people (especially teens) are very careless when it comes to eye examinations. This is exceptionally true for those who don't have a visual condition or those who don't wear glasses for distant vision.

You require periodic examination if:

- You have a driver's license
- You ride a bike (or have your own means of transportation)
- If you have any history of visual conditions in your family
- If you have any medical or autoimmune illnesses (like rheumatoid arthritis, hypertension, or diabetes)

Primarily in every eye examination, the healthcare provider performs vision analysis to check if eyesight is weak or not. This is followed by the doctor putting some drops in your eyes to enlarge the pupil, which provides the physician a better view to analyze the eye internally. This examination can be conducted using a slit lamp, which is a type of microscope that views the front of our eyes.

With the help of this slit lamp, inflamed cells and eye pressure can be judged. An eye exam is painless and is not as time consuming as one might expect. The dilatory effects will persist for six to twenty four hours, but this is nothing to worry about.

DENTAL HEALTH

Why is dental hygiene important?

To prevent gum diseases:

Gum diseases also called periodontitis, is an infection of the tooth/teeth. Bacteria on our teeth form plaque, which on hardening forms a black spot called tartar. If this condition is not stopped, teeth and mouth diseases can result.

Tooth loss:

When bacteria are not removed from the teeth properly, they start penetrating the skin where the tooth grows and cause damage to the roots. This damage can cause teeth to eventually loosen.

Smile:

Who doesn't want a perfect smile! Individuals can have stained teeth. This can be due to tobacco or medications, so a regular trip to the dentist will ensure a bright smile.

Mouth Odor:

Bad breath can be a sign of bad oral hygiene. This can be due to improper cleaning of teeth, infections, or bad eating habits. In this case, one must regularly clean their teeth and visit a dentist regularly.

Complete package:

Oral hygiene is also a part of our general hygiene. Evidence suggests that some oral diseases are related to other organ diseases. Therefore, constant and vigorous maintenance of our teeth is important to prevent not just oral, but other organ diseases from occurring.

Save money!

Keeping good oral health and regular checkups can help catch a disease in its early stages and can save money by avoiding the need of expensive and painful procedures, such as root canals, crowns, and dental implants.

What Is the Right Way to Brush?

Brush for at least two minutes, that's 120 seconds. I know that may seem long and most youth (and even adults) don't! Use short, gentle strokes, paying extra attention to your gumline, back teeth, and hard-to-reach areas.

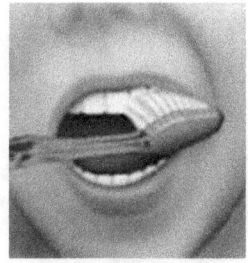
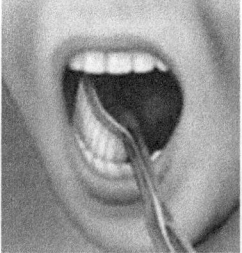
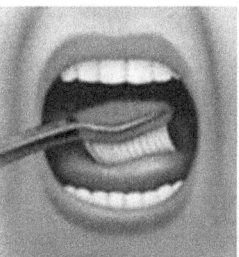

Tilt the brush at a 45° angle against the gumline and sweep or roll the brush away from the gumline.

Gently brush the outside, inside and chewing surface of each tooth using short back-and-forth strokes.

Gently brush your tongue to remove bacteria and freshen breath.

Self-Assessment for Chapter 2

- What are the benefits of periodic physical, ophthalmological, and dental examinations?
- What are common health issues that can be prevented by periodic examinations?
- How can you optimize your health by visiting your medical provider on a routine basis?

CHAPTER 3
REPRODUCTIVE HEALTH

Reproduction is a part of life and there are a number of facts and factors that teens are mostly unaware of. The aim of this chapter is to provide you a brief orientation to improve your understanding of teen reproduction and reproductive health.

Highlights of this Chapter:

- *Female Puberty*
- *Male Puberty*
- *Hygiene*
- *Menstruation*
- *Sex Education*
- *Sexual Transmitted Infections (STIs)*
- *HIV/AIDS*
- *Infertility*
- *Teen Pregnancy*
- *Contraceptives and Condoms*
- *Birth Control Methods*
- *Abstinence*

FEMALE PUBERTY

Puberty is the transformation to adulthood and during this period, several changes occur in the body, including the development and growth of sex organs. This is a confusing phase for certain people, while others enjoy this phase and feel proud. At the onset of puberty, the hypothalamus allows the pituitary gland to release gonadotropins hormones into the bloodstream. The body prepared this hormone a year before puberty starts. These hormones increase the production of estrogen (which is approximately 6 times more than pervious production) and production of androgen (which is approximately 20 times more than pervious production) in girl's ovaries and boy's testes, respectively.

Changes in females

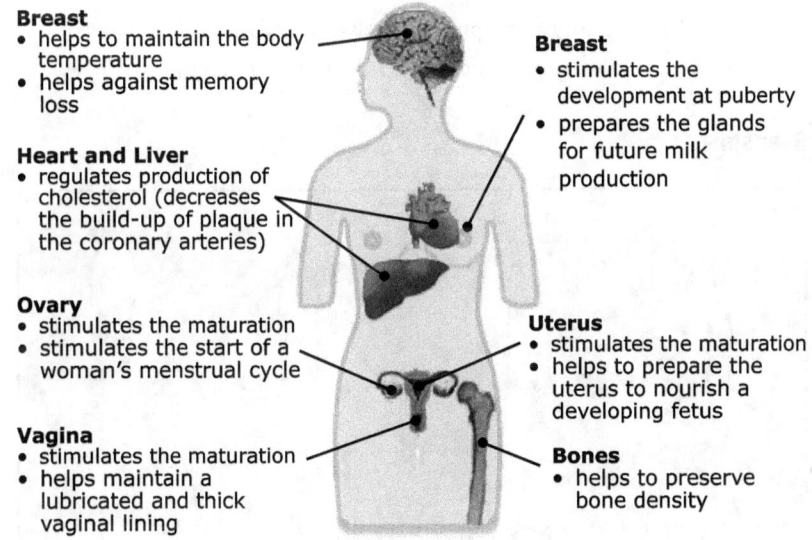

Effects of Estrogen

Breast
- helps to maintain the body temperature
- helps against memory loss

Heart and Liver
- regulates production of cholesterol (decreases the build-up of plaque in the coronary arteries)

Ovary
- stimulates the maturation
- stimulates the start of a woman's menstrual cycle

Vagina
- stimulates the maturation
- helps maintain a lubricated and thick vaginal lining

Breast
- stimulates the development at puberty
- prepares the glands for future milk production

Uterus
- stimulates the maturation
- helps to prepare the uterus to nourish a developing fetus

Bones
- helps to preserve bone density

During puberty, hibernating hormones suddenly wake up and signal the body to change. The time period of puberty varies from person to person. It can begin between age 8 to age 13 and be completed in a year or six years. During this period, several changes occur, including breast development, physical maturation, etc. Girls mature faster than boys. The reason behind this is that they enter puberty two years earlier than boys. The chart below outlines the time that physical changes occur during puberty.

Puberty Event	Age at which it occurs
Breast growth	Age 8 to 13
Pubic hair growth	Age 8 to 14
Body Growth	Age 9 ½ to 14 ½
First Period	Age 10 to 16 ½

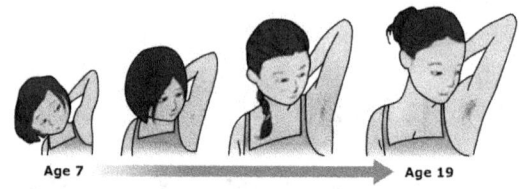

Underarm hair grows approximately 2 years after pubic hair. Acne occurs around the same time underarm hair grows.

Breasts

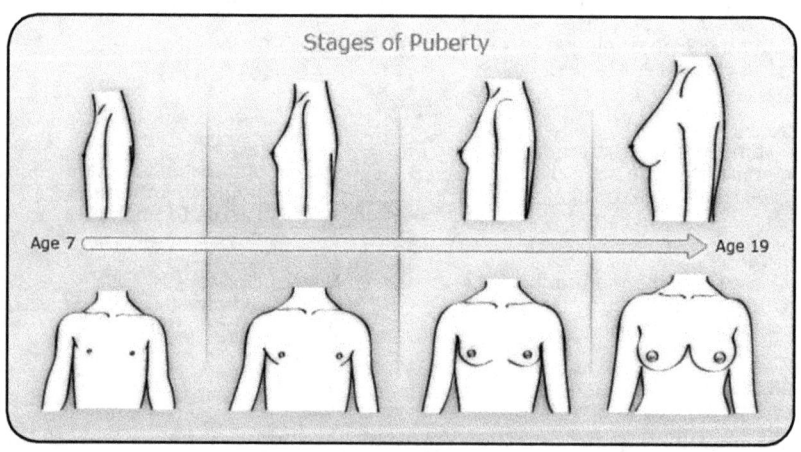

The breast start to develop from the flat area around the areola (nipple) which becomes enlarged and several tissues also form under the areola. After the completion of breast development, the areola doesn't appear as swollen.

Pubic Hair

Pubic hair grows at the vaginal lips and it becomes coarser and darker during puberty. It is also seen that pubic hair spread to thighs as well.

Growing

Puberty also gives a growth spurt and as a result a person grows 3.5 inches in a year. The first obvious things noticed are hands, head, and feet. Then the legs and arms grow, and lastly the shoulders and torso catch up with the remaining body parts. During puberty, weight gain is normal and without this weight a female cannot develop her breasts, get her first period, and grow taller.

Acne

During puberty the hair grows in the underarms, while sweat and glands that produce oil are also developed. When the glands get clogged, it results in acne. Washing your face twice daily helps prevent breakouts.

Menstruation:

Cindy was feeling a little weird for the last couple of months. She just celebrated her twelfth birthday with her friends and has always been a happy child. Yet for the last few weeks, she feels sad and depressed all the time. Her family and friends are also having a difficult time understanding her mood swings and edginess.

Are you aware that these symptoms (along with a few others that you will read about shortly) are normal according to Cindy's age?

As you have learned from the previous paragraphs, females experience puberty any time after their 11th birthday (or even earlier in some cases). Menstruation is an important part of the puberty phase that marks the "official" beginning of the fertility period.

What causes menstruation?

Every female is born with about 5 million eggs. However, these eggs remain in a static phase until she reaches puberty. At this time, female ovaries release tremendous amount of estrogen and other puberty hormones.

In response to the rising FSH (follicular stimulating hormone) release from a small gland in the brain, the ovaries begin to prepare a few eggs. However, only one egg survives, outgrows all other eggs, and is released into the fallopian tubes (small tubes that are connected to the ovaries). At the same time, female hormones also prepare the uterus (a pear-shaped organ in your pelvis that grows significantly to accommodate the baby in the event of pregnancy).

While the egg is in the tubes, if a sperm gains access to the tubes (via intercourse), the sperm and egg unite to form a zygote that can give rise to a baby. However, if no sperm comes in contact with the egg, the egg slowly degenerates.

At the same time, the uterine walls also begin to disintegrate and shed, leading to menstrual bleeding.

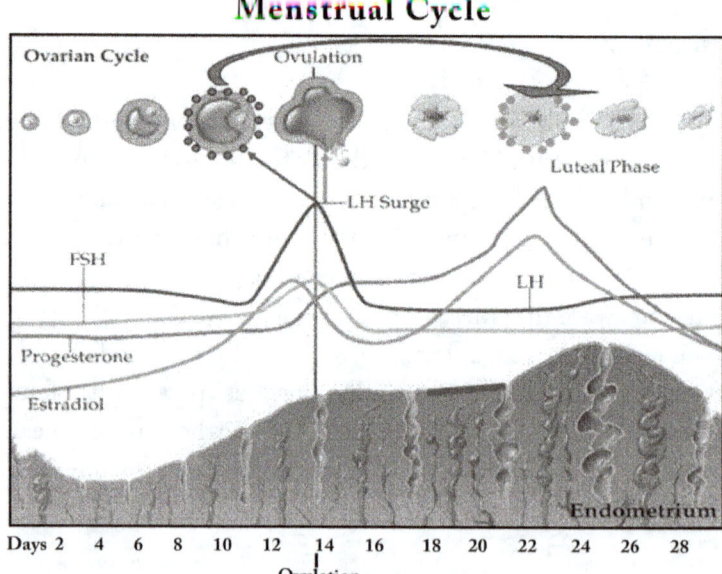

The egg is released into the fallopian tubes on the 14th day of the cycle; the lining begins to disintegrate during the third week (after 21 days) and bleeding occurs by the 28th day of the ovarian cycle (which is also considered as the first day of the menstrual cycle).

Menstruation is marked by these classic symptoms:

- Swelling or heaviness of breast (that may cause a dull feeling of soreness in some females)
- Mood swings
- Lower abdominal pain (dull aching in nature that may also involve the thighs, belly, and pelvic region). About 1-3% of females experience severe disabling pain that may require medications or other forms of therapy to alleviate..
- Passage of blood (or clots); the blood flow is usually high in the first couple of days and gradually decreases (and eventually fades out completely by day five to seven).
- Some females also experience bowel dysfunction (constipation or diarrhea).
- You may also experience a flaring in acne at the time of menstruation.

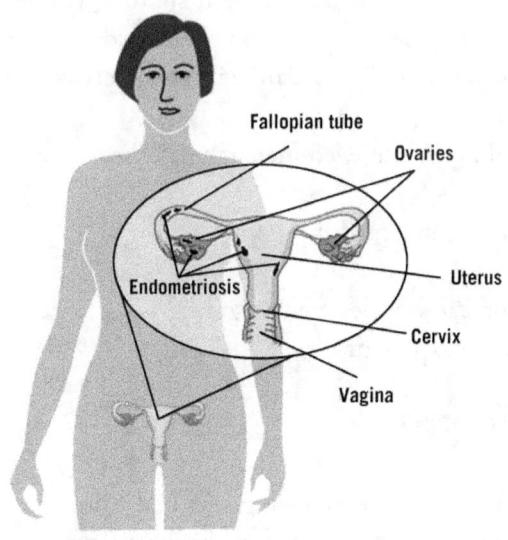

What can you do about it?

- Speak to your mother, female teacher, medical provider, or someone who can help you and address your main concerns
- Maintain optimal physical and reproductive hygiene
- Use sanitary pads and change at frequent intervals (avoid tampons, as minor carelessness can increase the risk of infections in female tampon users)
- Drink plenty of warm fluids and take an over-the-counter pain medication to manage pain (such as acetaminophen or ibuprofen)
- You can also use alternative therapies (such as massage, hydrotherapy, etc.) for pain relief.

Areas of Concern:

You should be concerned if:

- You are experiencing heavy bleeding with or without clots (more than 2 soaked pads in a period of 3 hours)
- If you are experiencing weakness, fatigue, dizziness
- If you are experiencing frequent spotting (in between cycles) or if your cycle length is less than 22 days or more than 35 days. Cycle length is the time interval between two menstrual cycles.
- If you haven't achieved menarche by the age of 15 years.

You shouldn't be concerned if:

- Your first few cycles aren't regular
- If you are experiencing mood swings

MALE PUBERTY

Hibernating hormones cause changes in male during puberty. It can begin from age 9 to age 13 ½ and this development is completed in 2 to 5 years. During this period, several changes occur, including growth of testicles, physical maturation, etc. The chart below outlines the time when physical changes occur in males during puberty.

Puberty Event	Age at which it happens
Testicles growth	Age 10 to 13 ½
Pubic hair growth	Age 10 to 15
Body Growth	Age 10 ½ to 16 ½
Penis growth	Age 11 to 14 ½
Voice change	Age 11 to 14 ½

Underarm hair grows approximately two years after pubic hair. Acne occurs around the same time underarm hair grows.

Genitalia & Pubic Hair

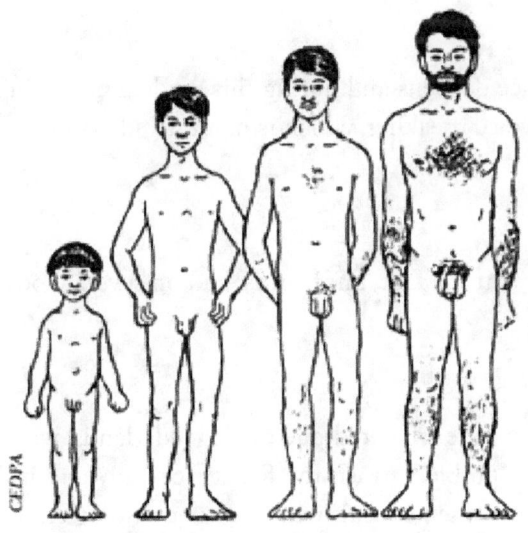

During early puberty stage, the scrotum enlarges with a change in the skin's texture. Pubic hair starts to appear at the base of the penis. The length of the penis increases with slight enhancement in width as well. The penis continues to grow until its head develops. The scrotum also grows and its skin becomes darker. After the development of the penis, you will notice pubic hair in an upside down position around the penis which spreads to thighs as well.

Growing

Puberty also causes a growth spurt and as a result a person grows 4.1 inches in a year. Firstly, the visible changes appear on the head, hands, and feet, then the legs and arms. Finally, the shoulders and torso catch up with remaining body parts.

Possible Breast Development

Some boys experience breast growth during puberty, which is temporary. It disappears after some time, however, if it doesn't, then consult with your doctor.

Voice Change

A male's voice deepens and during this gradual process a male might experience voice breaking, which is natural and normal.

Body Hair

Hair appears on the face, underarms, and on several body parts.

Acne

Acne problems are triggered due to clogged glands, which is natural. To avoid this problem, wash the face twice daily and if the problem becomes severe, then consult with your dermatologist.

PERSONAL HYGIENE

Below is some advice related to a teen's personal hygiene.

Baths and showers: it is important to take a bath every day and clean your body. When a child grows up and becomes a teenager, the body also experiences several changes which make it necessary for the teenager to pay extra attention towards personal hygiene. This means taking a shower daily. While taking a shower, clean the body with soap and then rinse it. The changes that occur in oil glands and sweat in teenagers make it vital to shower daily. Bad odor also comes from certain people, which is natural in the growing process. Washing the body with mild soap helps in cutting down odor and nabs that bacterium which causes the unpleasant smell.

Antiperspirant and deodorant:

If a teenager is annoyed with the smell factor and sweat, then use an antiperspirant and deodorant. Antiperspirant has the ability to dry the sweat glands, which further stops sweating and deodorant replaces the bad smell with the fragrance of flowers, baby powders, etc. A combination of both products is also available, and this consequently works best.

Hair care:

At the time of puberty, everything in the body starts to change, including hair. You may feel your scalp and hair become oily, requiring you to wash them more often. This is also a natural process and occurs due to hormonal changes in the body.

The hair texture of every girl is different, so there are several ways to take care of your hair. Some girls need to wash hair once a week, whereas some girls wash their hair daily to keep it from getting oily. This totally depends on a girl's genes, which no one can control. It is important to select hair care products that suits you and work best for you. The problem of oily hair can be control by washing hair daily, as washing cleans the oil from the hair and scalp. Use a mild shampoo and warm water for washing hair.

Dry hair needs a different type of care as compared to oily hair. Dry hair can damaged easily if you use the wrong shampoo or wash your hair daily. A good conditioner and a mild moisturizing shampoo can soften dry hair and make it more manageable.

Shaving:

Hair growing on different body parts is also another issue in youth that should be addressed. For shaving, seek the help of your mother, father, or any adult and take their advice related to shaving.

Some additional pieces of advice are:

- Use a good shaving cream that sooths the skin rather than irritating it.
- If you have sensitive skin, there are specially designed brands available for this skin type.
- Use a razor which is easy to utilize and can be controlled comfortably.
- While shaving legs, it is best to pull from the foot up.
- Take care while shaving around the ankles and knees, as the skin is bumpy there and you can easily cut yourself.
- Another way of removing hair is through waxing, but be careful while doing any procedure as it can irritate the skin. Therefore, consult with your dermatologist about your skin type and follow their advice.

INFERTILITY

As an adolescent, Samantha (Sammy) was a very casual girl, especially in terms of the relationships. She dated many boys and got in lots of troubles too.

She is now 24 and has been in a serious relationship for the last two years. Things are great and just like she always wanted, but there is one small problem. Despite her conscious attempts for the last four years, she hasn't been able to conceive.

Mark, Sammy's 28-year-old boyfriend, love kids and wants to start a family as early as possible. Sammy's think she might be infertile and wants to know why.

Female infertility is a common problem. Approximately 11% of all females encounter difficulty in becoming pregnant. But are all 11% actually infertile? Definitely not, since approximately 40% to 50% of females thought to be infertile actually become pregnant with simple education, diet and lifestyle modification, and learning more about the normal ovarian cycle.

What happens to remaining 6-7%?

This is a big chunk of the female population (in the reproductive age group), and the good news is that most females actually conceive with simple treatments and interventions

What may have caused infertility in Sammy's case?

There may be plenty of reasons. The most important and relevant factors are discussed in the pie chart below.

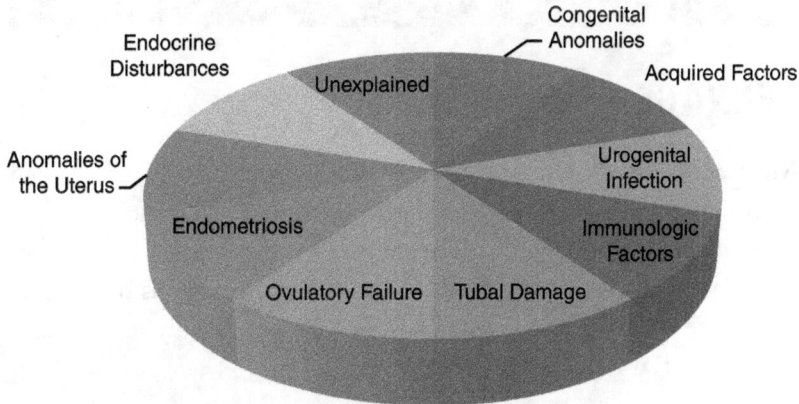

But it is also possible that her boyfriend Mark is infertile.

What can possibly cause infertility in males? Is it even a common cause of infertility?

Yes indeed!

Are you aware that in among 33% of all the reported cases of infertility, a defect or discrepancy in the male reproductive system is responsible for failure to impregnate the female partner? In another 33%, a primary defect in the female partner is responsible for an inability to get pregnant; whereas in the remaining 33%, a combined defect is responsible for infertility.

Knowing the possible causes of male infertility helps individuals and couples to seek early treatment.

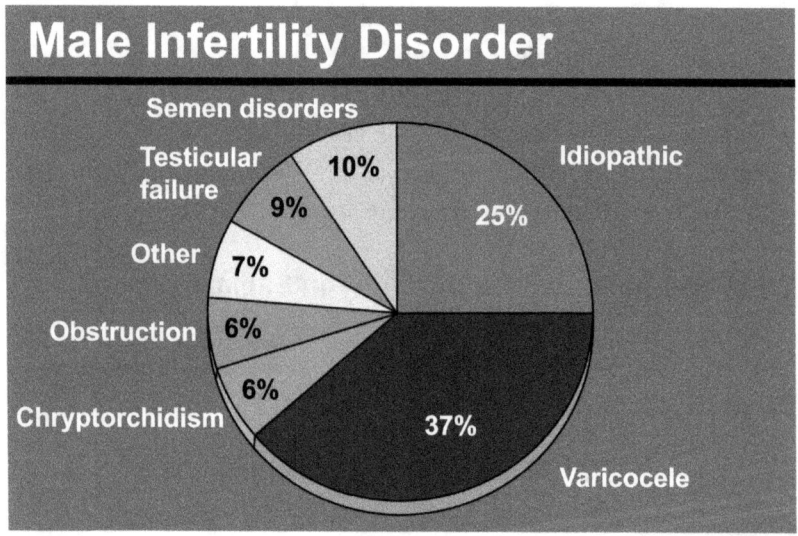

TEENAGE PREGNANCY

Most people spend their teen years being reckless and carefree about their actions, which directly affects their future. One such scenario is teenage pregnancy, which results when teens do not practice precaution, and as a result an infant becomes the responsibility of an immature set of parents. This practice is economically and socially non-beneficial for society.

Surveys suggest that teenage pregnancy lead to one or most of the following case scenarios: dropping out of high school, economic crisis, increase in depression and suicide rates, risk to personal health, and most dangerous of all, risk of STDs (Sexually Transmitted Diseases).

Hazards of teenage pregnancy

Most teen mothers are not fully mature physically, hence giving birth to a baby is not only a danger to the child, it is also a direct danger to the mother. Furthermore, the chances of a malnourished child are increased considerably. If the mother is infected with a disease, she may pass it on to the child, resulting in a deformed, undeveloped child or one with a high mortality rate.

Oftentimes, young females are more careless towards their health and are more likely to make reckless decisions that may lead to the death of the baby or their own death. In other cases, careless behavior may lead to legal issues and may destroy the life of a teen, as happened with Rennie.

Teen Mom Used Cocaine While Pregnant. Her Baby Died. Mississippi Charged Her With Murder

In 2006, Mississippi teenager Rennie Gibbs gave birth to a little girl, Samiya, who was born a month premature. Gibbs arrived at the hospital with a stillborn baby whose umbilical cord was wrapped around her neck. Gibbs was indicted for murder shortly thereafter, and has spent the previous seven years fighting for her release. The indictment was a result of a highly controversial forensic examiner named Steven Hayne, who found in the baby's blood traces of benzoylecgonine, a cocaine byproduct. He declared that the baby's cause of death was maternal cocaine use. (No actual cocaine was found in Samiya's body.) ProPublica representative Nina Martin commented on the case, putting it in the context of the larger nationwide push to hold women, especially young women of color, criminally accountable for failing to produce a live baby when they give birth.

How to avoid teen pregnancy?

To avoid teenage pregnancy, teenagers should practice caution with protection, limit sexual partners to avoid disease transmission, and furthermore seek a physician's advice for any health problems after intercourse, which can help protect them from any predisposed diseases.

It is never too late.

Upon finding out about the pregnancy, a teenager should immediately take certain steps.

- She should consult a doctor immediately, and receive education about her options.
- She should speak to her parents (or guardian) and partner about it.
- Educate herself about childbirth and child rearing.
- Try and manage financial matters.
- Adopt a healthy lifestyle by quitting unhealthy habits like drinking and smoking.
- Exercise on a regular basis and maintain a healthy diet.

HIV (HUMAN IMMUNODEFICIENCY VIRUS)

They say it is better to be safe than sorry, and HIV/AIDS is one such case where some caution and prevention can not only save lives, but also prevent turmoil in a society.

HIV/AIDS, also known as Human Immunodeficiency Virus/Acquired Immunodeficiency Syndrome, is a viral disease that gradually destroys the body's immune system, making it vulnerable to other diseases.

The statistics regarding this disease are not only staggering, but also highlight the importance of how critical it is to control and prevent this disease. In the US, about 50,000 new cases are reported each year. The incidence of HIV is higher amongst African Americans and approximately two-third of all new cases reported are bi-sexual individuals.

What is HIV?

The HIV virus attacks the immunity of a body, making it weak and susceptible to other infections. The immune system is our armor against disease causing pathogens, so the lack of it can lead to death from the least life threatening infections, such as the flu, fever, minor bacterial attacks, and even the common cold.

The initial symptoms a person faces include nausea, flu, cough, vomiting, recurrent pain, weight loss, etc.

As the disease progresses, the signs and symptoms become more severe. They include systemic fungal infections, chronic ulcers, chronic body pains, chronic cough, and blisters and sores on odd areas of their body.

Transmission of HIV

Transmission of HIV is different from other diseases. It does not spread via touch or through the air, but the disease is transmitted by fluid exchange. This can include blood, semen, or sputum exchange with an infected individual.

Man sentenced in HIV assault

A Waco man was sentenced to 40 years after he had unprotected sex with three young teens and transmitted the deadly virus to two of them. Thirty-nine-year-old Dennis Germaine Nobles was sentenced to 40 years in prison after he plead guilty to two counts of sexual assault of a child, three counts of assault-family violence and two counts of aggravated assault with a deadly weapon.

Nobles was charged in the case as a habitual criminal because of his extensive criminal background, which includes three prior felonies and 10 misdemeanor convictions.

He pleaded guilty to having intercourse in 2010 with a 17-year-old girl and a 16-year-old girl. According to records filed in the case, the 17-year-old became infected with the human immunodeficiency virus, but the younger girl did not.

Nobles faced a minimum sentence of 25 years and maximum term of life in prison before accepting the plea agreement that will keep him in prison for at least 20 years.

He is charged with aggravated assault with a deadly weapon (since he was aware of his HIV status, but still decided to have unprotected sexual activities).

One of the girls was younger than 17, which is why the sexual assault counts were filed.

Nobles also pleaded guilty to charges of assault directed against his stepdaughter and wife.

Source: http://www.wacotrib.com/news/courts_and_trials/man-sentenced-in-hivassault/article_e47c0c96-6973-59be-b678-c84848060ec4.html

---

Transmission can occur in three basic modes. The first way is vertical, that is passing of the disease from mother to baby. Second is through sexual contact, and third is through infected needles.

High-risk groups

As research shows, drug addicts and bisexuals are the most high-risk groups. Besides these, sex workers (prostitutes), polygamous individuals, and people with a history of STDs/STIs (sexually transmitted infections/sexually transmitted infections) are also at high risk of not only acquiring the disease, but also spreading it to others.

HIV treatment

The spread of this disease is very quick and silent. It is critical that HIV be diagnosed as early as possible so that treatment can begin. There are drugs/medications available today, such as Anti-retroviral drugs, that enable HIV to be managed effectively. If HIV is prevented from becoming full-blown AIDS, a person can expect to live a long life, although there is no cure. By the time HIV turns into AIDS, the body is practically incapable of recovering. AIDS completely destroys the immune system. As a result, people end up dying from things like the flu, pneumonia, or even the common cold.

Preventing HIV

We now have more information regarding the prevention of HIV than curing it. There are many ways which are simple yet crucial in keeping away from this life threatening and ultimately fatal disease. They include:

- Using protection for sexual interaction.
- Know your sexual partner well—that is know that they are STD free and are healthy individuals.
- Use new needles, fresh from a sterile pack every time.
- Avoid using contaminated needles even among family members.
- Have your partner get tested if you observe signs of illness or spots over their body.
- On exposure to the infection, rush to the hospital to get tested and treated.

CONTRACEPTIVES AND BIRTH CONTROL METHODS

CONDOMS

It is one of the cheapest forms of contraception. A condom is a thin cover which wraps around the penis while engaged in intercourse. Condoms are made from latex (rubber), lambskin, or polyurethane (plastic). Male condoms are available in different sizes, color, and quantity of spermicide and lubrication.

Condoms have the capacity to prevent pregnancy and STIs (sexually transmitted infections) by covering the penis and prevent exchange of bodily fluids. The latex condom has the capacity to protect against STIs such as HIV. Plastic condoms also protect against several infections but are not as effective as latex. However, lambskin condoms, while able to prevent pregnancy, cannot protect against several STIs and HIV. Condoms also collect semen and keep it from entering the vagina.

How is it used?

The condom is placed at the tip (or head) of an erect or hardened penis, then completely rolled down the shaft of the penis. It prevents the direct contact of the vagina and the penis. The condom should be immediately removed, after sex and before the penis becomes soft, to prevent sperm from leaking out into the vagina. Always use condom once and throw it into the garbage after use. Don't flush condoms down the toilet, and NEVER use a condom more than once.

Condoms protect against unwanted teenage pregnancy

Condoms, in conjunction with spermicide, help in preventing pregnancy. For achieving best results, use condom before the sperm or pre-ejaculate comes in contact with the vagina. With typical use of a condom (latex), there is only a 14% chance that a female can get pregnant, whereas with perfect use of a condom (latex), there is only a 3% chance of pregnancy.

Advantages of condom:

- Can be attained easily and doesn't require any prescription
- It is best for preventing STIs and several other infections
- Preventing an unwanted pregnancy and protects both partners against several sexually transmitted diseases (STIs).

What should you know about Condoms?

- Some people are allergic to latex. They can use polyurethane condoms as an alternative.
- Many people reported that using condoms decreases pleasure and sensitivity during intercourse.
- Some people don't like interrupting sex to put them on.
- Condoms can break if not used correctly.

Things to Remember

The following are important things you should know prior to using condoms.

- A female condom can't be used in combination with a male condom
- Avoid using latex condoms with any oil-based lubricants, including Vaseline, petroleum jelly, or vegetable and mineral oil. These lubricants can damage the condom or cause it to break.
- Condoms should be guarded from heat, especially latex condoms. Heat can break the condom or can weaken it.
- Condoms have expiration dates. Once this date has passed, the condom is too weak to provide effective protection.

What are some other methods of contraception?

There are several aims and objectives of practicing contraception. Not only do these small measures prevent unwanted pregnancy, but also help in reducing the risk of STIs.

You can choose your contraceptive device after careful consideration of your aims and objectives. Below is a chart that describes the effectiveness and benefits of using each method.

Temporary Contraception

These methods provide temporary contraception (which means a pregnancy is possible if you stop using these methods). Permanent contraceptive methods render a male or female infertile or sterile (which means no pregnancy is possible after having these procedures done).

	Abstinence	Fertility Awareness Method (FAM)	Spermicide	Condom	Diaphragm/ Cervical Cap
What it is?	A decision to avoid harmful behaviors, such as sex, alcohol, and drugs	Methods of contraceptives that determine the female cycle	A chemical that kills sperm	Thin sheath of latex, plastic, or animal tissue that is placed on the penis to catch semen	A latex cup with flexible rim that covers the cervix
How does it work?	Abstain from sexual activity until marriage	Involves a female taking temperature every morning or checking the mucus of the cervix	Coats condom to help kill sperm	Rolled onto erect penis before sex	A physical barrier to the passage of sperm
Advantages	It is the only 100% effective method in preventing pregnancy and disease	Helps to reduce unwanted pregnancy	Helps to prevent unwanted pregnancy	Helps prevent STIs/STDs and unwanted pregnancy	Helps to prevent unwanted pregnancy

Disadvantages	NONE	-Doesn't prevent STIs/STDs - Not 100% effective, only 80% effective	Not always effective	May break, not 100% effective	Not always effective
Side Effects	NONE	Unwanted pregnancy	Unwanted pregnancy	-An STI/STD -Unwanted pregnancy	Pregnancy
Where can you get it from?	YOURSELF	Must consult a healthcare professional	-Healthcare professionals -Drug stores -Condoms may also have it	-Drug stores -School -Health Dept.	Your healthcare professional

Besides the previous commonly used methods, there are also permanent methods.

	Vasectomy	**Tubal Ligation**
What it is?	A sterile procedure for males	A sterilization procedure for females
How does it work?	The Vas Deferens is cut so sperm will not enter seminal stream (ejaculate)	The fallopian tubes are tied or clamped to prevent sperm from reaching ovum
Advantages	Procedure is 99.9% effective	Procedure is 99.9% effective
Disadvantages	- Does not protect against STDs - Can't have children - Reversal is expensive	- Does not protect against STDs - Can't be reversed

Side Effects	Prevents the male from releasing sperm	Cramps, heavier bleeding, pelvic bleeding
Where can you have it done?	Doctor who specializes in it	Doctor who specializes in it

ABSTINENCE

It has been observed that one of the leading causes of abortions, high school dropouts, poor academic performance in schools, and inclination to use drugs and alcohol is unplanned pregnancy. There are a number of methods that can be used to prevent teenage pregnancy.

The overall prevalence of teenage pregnancy is on the rise. Inadequate knowledge about contraception can also lead to further complications, such as improper child spacing, poor maternal and child health, and economic turmoil that further push teens to violence and crimes to earn easy money in order to support their child. Obviously, any such situation can further increase the risk of a strained parent-child relationship. Practicing adequate and safe contraception is a desirable strategy to prevent all these problems, but unfortunately a lot of teens are either unaware of contraception methods or don't want to practice them because of a lack of complete knowledge and potential benefits.

But there is something else that teens should consider.

Sexual intercourse at a young age is associated with a higher risk of several complications and issues such as sexually transmitted diseases, an increased risk to develop cervical cancer in females (that is directly related to the age at first intercourse), and several other ailments.

To restrain from engaging in sexual activities is perhaps the only method that may provide absolute risk-free prevention from teenage pregnancy. Besides, if you are a teenager looking for effective contraceptive methods, you should know that most commonly employed contraceptive devices or products carry hazards associated with long-term use (such as abruption of normal biochemical rhythm and weight gain in case of oral contraceptives; pelvic inflammatory disease, inflammation and infection of the pelvic tract in cases of IUDs and so forth).

On the contrary, abstinence has several other benefits as well.

What are some of the benefits of abstinence?

> ### Abstinence gives you freedom! FREEDOM from:
> - Guilt or dishonesty to oneself or family
> - Loss of future goals or plans
> - Sexually transmitted diseases
> - Unwanted pregnancy
> - Difficult abortion or adoption decision
> - Negative reputation
> - Birth control side effects
> - Broken heart or rejection

Isn't it pretty hard to leave some of the most fun stuff and activities during teenage years! It is definitely hard to resist the charm and fun that most of the movies and today's television dramas show, such as sex, drugs, fun, partying, and adventure. But I must warn you that the prevalence of sexually transmitted diseases (STI's) in teens is on the rise. The reason for this is unprotected sexual intercourse.

What else should you know?

Of course abstinence is an effective method for preventing unwanted teen pregnancy and sexually transmitted diseases, yet it is very important that you still know about safe sex and other aspects of sexual education. Some studies suggested that with prolonged abstinence (especially in teens who have had a sexual encounter before), the risk of chance encounters increases significantly.

The risk of getting pregnant is equally high if no abstinence is practiced. A lot of teens feel extremely troubled and stressed out after becoming pregnant; knowing there are extremely few options for them brings a lot of stress, agitation, and agony. Most teens end up doing stuff they never expected or wanted.

Here is an example of a young teen pregnant female who got so stressed out that she ended up assaulting a bus driver. Needless to say, she is very likely to face criminal charges.

Pregnant teen assault bus driver due to fare dispute

According to police sources, pregnant teen Natasha Lawson, 19, assaulted an MTA bus driver on a Brooklyn bus this Saturday morning. She boarded the bus between Troy Avenue and Kings Highway somewhere around 7:30 a.m. However, she was short of the fare by $1.75. After failing to strike a bargain with bus driver Jenny Castillo, Lawson requested Castillo to take her halfway, to Nostrand Avenue. However, when the driver (who is 36) refused, the pregnant teen boldly strode to the back of the bus and began to harass the elderly passengers, according to MTA sources.

Castillo tried to stop Lawson and ordered her to get off the bus, sources said. That's when the three months pregnant teen punched and scratched Castillo in the face and pulled her hair, police sources said. Riders held the mom-to-be down as cops responded to the assault in progress, police sources reported.

Castillo was treated for superficial injuries at Beth Israel Hospital and Lawson was admitted for psychiatric evaluation at the same hospital.

http://nypost.com/2014/03/22/pregnant-teen-assaults-bus-driver-in-fare-dispute/

Self-Assessment for Chapter 3

- What are some potential hazards of teenage pregnancy?
- How can you prevent teenage pregnancy?
- What are some effective methods of contraception?
- What are some benefits of condoms and contraceptives?
- How can you minimize the transmission of sexually transmitted diseases?
- Why is HIV so bad? How can you prevent the infection?
- What is abstinence?
- What are some benefits of waiting until you're married to have sex?
- What is infertility?

CHAPTER 4
COMMON CHRONIC DISEASES IN YOUTH

Highlights of this Chapter

The aim of this chapter is to discuss some common health issues that most teens face. In addition to physiological or medical illnesses, this chapter will also help to explain the management options and how to cope with these illnesses.

- *Obesity*
- *Asthma*
- *Juvenile Diabetes*
- *Acne*

COMMON CHRONIC DISEASES IN YOUTH

Being a child or an adolescent is indeed the most fun part of your lifetime. Believe it or not, with age, things get tough and more challenging. Oftentimes, when we are dealing with something harsh like a chronic illness or disease, it directly affects our morale and energy levels.

- *Is it normal?*
- *Is it helpful?*
- *And more importantly is there a mature solution?*

The answer to the first question is YES! Yes, you may feel low at times in the face of chronic health issues, but there are always mature and productive solutions that may help you to live a near-normal and functional life.

How can you do that?

Diseases, illnesses, and health issues are a part of life. Situations are different if you have chronic health issues. Chronic diseases are medical problems that may take a longer time to resolve completely. In some cases (like juvenile diabetes and asthma), the health issue may be lifelong, but with proper management, symptoms can be controlled.

Educate yourself about health issues

It is a common observation that due to the longer course of illness, chronic diseases are often hard to deal with. You may have to visit your healthcare professional more frequently for medical evaluation or management of emergencies.

If you have a chronic health condition, it is very important to seek knowledge and learn about your condition to:

- Prevent or delay complications
- Maintain optimal health
- Minimize emergency care visits
- Live a normal life like your peers

What are some common chronic health issues in youth?

Do not think that you are alone. A recent survey suggested that one of every two Americans have at least one health issue. The ideal approach to deal with this situation is to look for remedies and solutions to prevent diseases and disorders.

The following are some chronic diseases that are fairly common in adolescents. There are other resources to learn more about these health issues.

OBESITY

According to a survey conducted by CDC (Center for Disease Control and Prevention), the overall rate of obesity is increasing at a very rapid pace in individuals of all age groups. Likewise, the percentage of overweight teens and children is also growing dramatically with every passing day.

Can you believe that one-third of the entire US population is obese?

The percentage of overweight youth has tripled since 1980. Furthermore, the data also suggests that 30% of teens and children belonging to age group 6 - 19 years are overweight

What is Obesity?

Excessive deposition of fat in the body is referred to as obesity. In sophisticated terms, body mass index (BMI) of 28 kg/m2 or more is classified as obesity *(please review the charts and tables below to learn how to calculate your BMI).*

$$\text{Body Mass Index} = \frac{\text{Weight (in kg)}}{\text{Height}^2 \text{ (in m)}}$$

BMI Chart

BMI less than 18.50	Underweight
BMI 18.50 - 24.99	Healthy weight
BMI 25.00 - 29.99	Overweight
BMI 30 or more	Obese

http://www.webmd.com/diet/calc-bmi-plus

An obese person is 20% heavier than their ideal or recommended body weight. Obesity is often associated with abnormal eating behavior that is fairly common in adolescence. The term overweight can be explained as having excess weight that is higher than the ideal limit range, or a body mass index of more than 25 kg/m2.

It was previously believed that adolescents or kids are less likely to develop health problems due to obesity as compared to adults. Yet the latest statistics suggests otherwise.

There is a 40% chance that an overweight child will grow into an overweight teenager, and an 80% chance that an overweight teenager will become an overweight or obese adult. And you will learn in the next section how dangerous obesity actually is.

Are you aware how the rate of obesity has grown over the past few decades?

Here is a close analysis…

Obesity rates have increased substantially over the past 20 years and are highest in the US

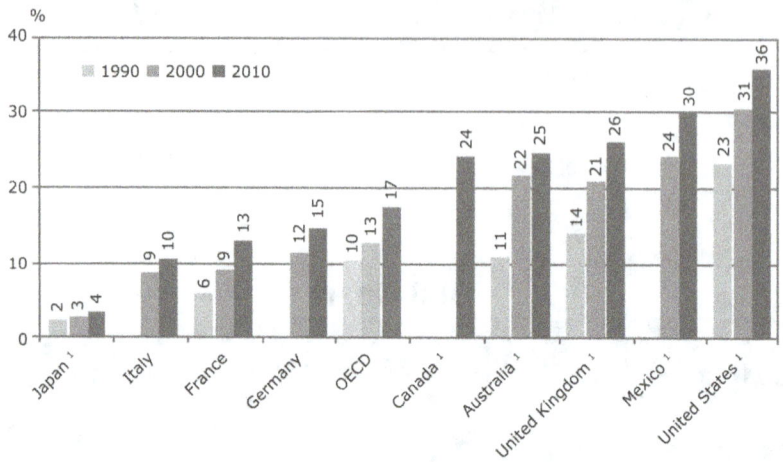

1. Data are based on measurements rather than self-reported height and weight.
Source: OECD Health Data 2012.

Why is BMI and obesity such a big deal?

You may feel that a high BMI or being obese is not that big of a deal. But the fact is, some serious health issues are directly associated with obesity, such as:

- Heart diseases
- High blood pressure
- Diabetes
- Several cancers
- Stroke

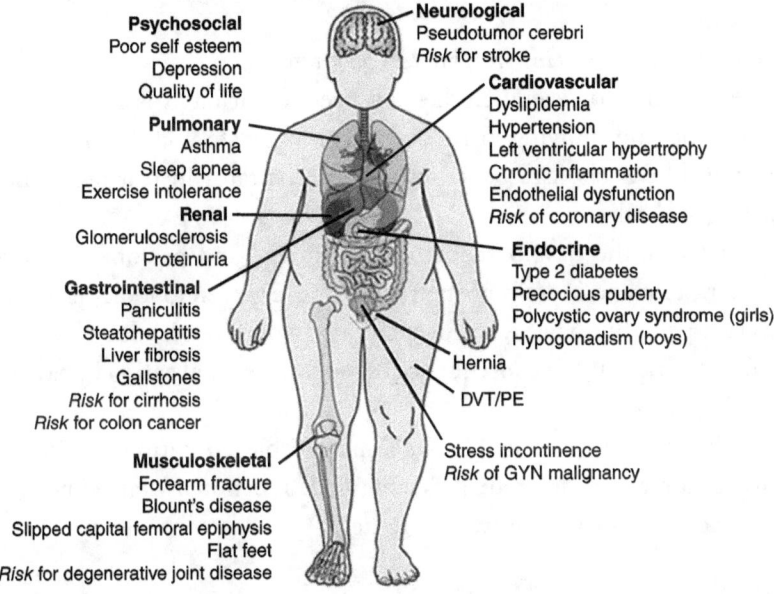

Complications of Childhood Obesity

Psychosocial
Poor self esteem
Depression
Quality of life

Pulmonary
Asthma
Sleep apnea
Exercise intolerance

Renal
Glomerulosclerosis
Proteinuria

Gastrointestinal
Paniculitis
Steatohepatitis
Liver fibrosis
Gallstones
Risk for cirrhosis
Risk for colon cancer

Musculoskeletal
Forearm fracture
Blount's disease
Slipped capital femoral epiphysis
Flat feet
Risk for degenerative joint disease

Neurological
Pseudotumor cerebri
Risk for stroke

Cardiovascular
Dyslipidemia
Hypertension
Left ventricular hypertrophy
Chronic inflammation
Endothelial dysfunction
Risk of coronary disease

Endocrine
Type 2 diabetes
Precocious puberty
Polycystic ovary syndrome (girls)
Hypogonadism (boys)

Hernia

DVT/PE

Stress incontinence
Risk of GYN malignancy

Obesity can destroy the overall well-being and physical health of a person and reduces overall life expectancy. Obesity can also cause unhappiness and social disabilities that further lead to stress and raise the risk of mental illness in teens.

What can you do about it?

Case # 1:

Karen has always been a chubby kid, but it was never a problem. Her family members and relatives call her "cute" and "pretty." But ever since she has started going to this new high school, she has been troubled.

Megan (Meg) and her group of friends call her names and make fun of her chubby appearance. **Karen** *is just so confused and to some extent embarrassed by her physical appearance. She read somewhere that the only solution for weight loss is reducing food intake to no more than 1 serving* *in the whole day. Her best friend also suggested purging as a possible substitute.*

Karen *is considering starting this behavior....*

According to several studies, an overweight child is more prone to teasing and bullying at school as compared to a child of normal weight. He or she can be a victim or perpetrator in teasing, name-calling, or bullying.

In teens, the development of body image and personal identity matters a lot and is an important goal for every teen to look perfect in every aspect. But what Karen is planning to do is not healthy. You will learn more about the consequences of such abnormal eating behaviors in Chapter 9.

Obesity is a preventable and manageable condition, ONLY if proper intervention or help is obtained. Do not use an abnormal behavior to manage your weight issues.

If you are obese or you are looking to lose weight:

- Talk to your parents, guardian, teacher, or someone you trust and express your desires and concerns.
- Speak to a medical provider, health coach, dietitian, or nutritionist to learn more about healthy nutrition and available options.
- Eliminate foods and beverages that contain high fructose corn syrup because they cause obesity and other health issues.
- Avoid processed foods, because they contain sodium, sugar, and unhealthy fats, and not enough nutrients.
- Cut down your caloric intake without altering your food intake. Starving your body increases weight gain in the future by decreasing your metabolism.
- Engage yourself in healthy behavior and activities. Sports and physical activity is the most important element in maintaining a healthy metabolism and body weight.

It is the duty of parents and teachers to help their children and take them to see a medical provider if necessary. An overweight child should talk to a parent/guardian or a person they trust for guidance related to health problems.

Activity:

Calculate your body mass index and see where your total body weight falls:

  a. Under-weight
  b. Normal
  c. Over-weight
  d. Obese

(Hint: You can confirm your results with the table located in the resources section at the back of the book. Also included is an easier method to calculate your BMI)

ASTHMA

Asthma is an allergic condition that primarily interferes with the respiratory system of an individual. During an asthma attack, the muscles around the airways become spastic or tight along the inner lining of airways. The resultant effect is swelling or thickening of respiratory passageways. In addition, due to an allergic response, the respiratory cells release heavy and thick mucus that further make gaseous exchange more difficult.

Here is a graphic explanation of what happens in an acute asthma attack.

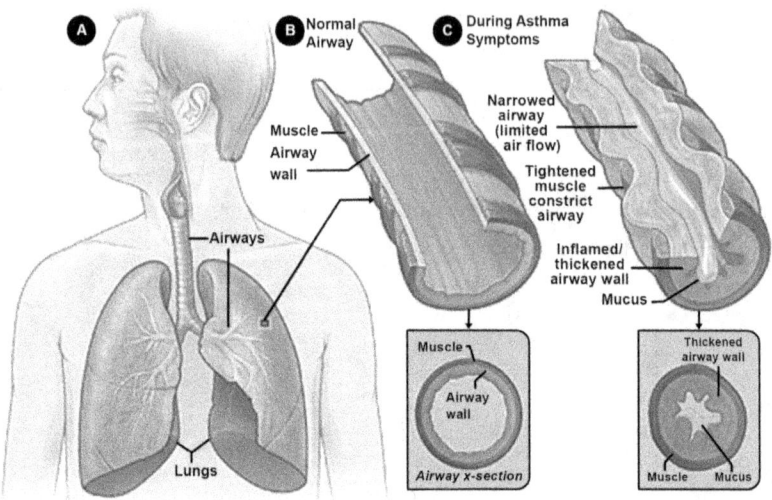

Figure A shows the location of the lungs and airways in the body. Figure B shows a cross-section of a normal airway. Figure C shows a cross-section of an airway during asthma symptoms.

Common Symptoms of Asthma

You may have all, some, or one of the following symptoms. Symptoms can be mild to severe.

- Coughing
- Wheezing (a whistling noise when you breath)
- Chest tightness (a feeling that your chest is squeezed or a feeling that someone is sitting on your chest)
- Shortness of breath

During an acute attack of asthma, the person may collapse, feel short of breath, and (in severe attacks) even die due to internal suffocation.

What may increase your risk of asthma?

Most adolescents develop some signs of asthma by their teen years. Although any person can develop asthma or allergic respiratory conditions, the risk increases significantly in these situations:

- Family history of asthma or any blood relative with active asthma
- History of other allergic conditions (like eczema)
- Babies born to mothers who smoke
- Low birth weight

What may trigger an asthma attack?

It is very important to understand that certain factors may induce or worsen an asthma attack. While there is little you can do to CURE asthma, you can definitely adopt some healthy interventions to minimize your risk of developing acute asthma attacks.

- Bronchitis or cold infections
- Changing weather
- Smoke and smoking
- Strenuous physical activity or severe exercise
- Pollen
- Dust mites
- Cats
- Obesity
- Stress
- Exposure to manufacturing chemicals, pollution, germs, or allergens.

Asthma attacks, if not addressed properly, can limit social activities and physical participation of a teen. However, with early identification, proper treatment, and incorporation of preventive options, you can live a normal life.

How can you manage your asthma?

Case # 2:

Jason, an athletic teen, has recently been discharged from the emergency center of the town hospital. He was admitted three days ago for the management of an acute asthma attack. Jason was diagnosed with asthma one year ago, and this was his 5th hospital admission since then.

Because of weakness and high frequency of admission to emergency centers, his academic performance is suffering, and he is hardly keeping up with his tough exercise routine.

- *His doctors have failed to understand the poor response to therapy. What are other factors that may be contributing to Jason's asthma attacks?*
- *Can he do anything to decrease the frequency of attacks and improve his academic performance?*

Jason's high frequency of attacks and poor response to therapy can be associated with his vigorous exercise routine. Proper warm-up and cool-down may prevent or reduce exercise-induced asthma. This chronic disease cannot be cured, but the symptoms are controllable. The following tips can help you in managing your asthma issues.

What do you think?

- Make an action plan with your doctor for managing your asthma problem. Write down all the medications that you consume for the management of asthma (both acute management and long-term preventive management). It is important to follow that plan because asthma conditions remains with you for life and its regular treatment and monitoring is necessary.
- It is important to get vaccinated against seasonal respiratory infections like pneumonia and influenza.
- Discover and identify the conditions that act as triggers of your asthma attacks or that make it worse. Try your best to avoid

such triggers. Oftentimes, you can also seek de-sensitization treatments to decrease the intensity of attacks.
- Observe your breathing and identify the warning signals of an imminent attack, such as wheezing, coughing, and shortness of breath. It is common that people do not notice the symptoms until it is too late.
- Observe and monitor the frequency of inhaler use. If you are using it more often, then your asthma might be resurfacing. Immediately discuss any changes with your medical provider to improve your condition and prevent serious complications.
- Continue taking medications, even if the asthma improves. Talk to your doctor before stopping any medications. It is also important to take the right dosage and correct medicine to avoid triggering asthma attacks.
- Treating an asthma attack early will require fewer medications and decrease the risk of a serious asthma attack. Whenever you notice the decline in peak flow measurement, immediately take the medications and avoid anything that triggers the attack.

TYPE 1 DIABETES (JUVENILE DIABETES)

According to the results of a survey conducted by the American Diabetes Association, six percent of the United States population is currently diabetic (that corresponds to 18 million adults). The report also suggested that only 13 million people are currently aware of or officially diagnosed as diabetics, while over 5 million individuals (one-third of the entire diabetic population) are unaware of the illness.

What is diabetes?

A disease in which the human body does not use or produce insulin (the key hormone that regulates sugar concentration in the blood) is termed as diabetes. This hormone plays an important role in converting starches, sugar, and several foods into energy, which is required by the human body at all times. The main cause of this metabolic disorder is not yet known. However, some factors such as genetics, lack of physical exercise, and obesity are recognized as risk factors.

What is juvenile diabetes and how is it different from adult diabetes?

- **Type 1** – also called insulin dependent diabetes, and previously known as Juvenile Diabetes, is usually reported in children or adolescents. In Type 1 diabetes, the body does not produce insulin at all. Consequently, the person requires insulin injections to maintain blood sugar levels within normal limits.
- **Type 2** – 90% of people in the world with diabetes suffer from Type 2 diabetes. Previously it was termed as maturity-onset or non-insulin dependent diabetes. The World Health Organization states that over 300 million people have Type 2 diabetes and their numbers are increasing rapidly. In Type 2 diabetes, insulin production is insufficient to perform the tasks required by the body. Obesity increases a person's risk of developing this type of diabetes. Being an adolescent, you are at a lesser risk of developing Type 2 diabetes, unless you are morbidly obese.

Why is it important to monitor blood sugar levels?

Isn't it hard to resist candies and stay away from chocolates and desserts?

It definitely is…. And if you are a Type 1 diabetic, you should know that managing your blood sugar levels is extremely important.

Uncontrolled or poorly managed diabetes can lead to disabling complications, such as:

- Stroke (due to damage to blood vessels supplying the brain tissue)
- Blindness/ vision loss
- Heart disease
- Kidney problems
- Poor wound healing, high risk of developing foot ulcers (if foot hygiene is not maintained), and in severe cases amputation may be needed.

That's why if you are a diabetic, you should take extra caution to maintain a normal blood sugar concentration.

What are some of the classic symptoms of diabetes?

Are you aware that diabetes is known as a "silent killer" since most of the symptoms are non-specific and slow to emerge. If you have a positive family history of diabetes or if you have other autoimmune diseases, take these symptoms very seriously and immediately report to your healthcare professional for emergent management:

- Persistent thirst (regardless of oral water intake, the thirst just doesn't go away)
- Feeling tired or weak (due to loss of all your dietary nutrients in urine)
- Too much urination (with a sweet musty smell and a sweet taste—*oh don't try to taste the urine, let the lab technicians do their job*)
- Abnormal weight loss
- Distorted vision
- Numbness or tingling in feet or hands
- Bruises and cuts that may take an unnecessary amount of time in healing

- Frequently occurring infections that may range from boils and furuncles to fungal and urinary tract infections (UTIs)
- Problems maintaining an erection in some males and abnormal vaginal dryness in some females
- Intense hunger
- Vomiting
- Feeling of being nauseated all the time

How can it affect your life?

Chronic diseases like diabetes may interfere with your productivity or stamina. You may not feel as energetic and vibrant as your peers, but always remember that:

- Proper nutritional guidance and support can help you live a normal life
- Maintain your blood sugar levels and keep up with your routine health examinations
- Consume low glycemic meals that do not cause a rapid spike in blood sugar levels.

Activity:

Can you name some low glycemic foods?

(Hint: See the end of this book to learn about low glycemic foods)

ACNE

We all notice and hate those red and pink bumps on our skin that leaves brown and black pigmentation or scars. Acne is a dermatological condition that is very well related to the hormonal changes of puberty and may cause a lot of stress for young adolescents.

The primary pathophysiological event is the accumulation of dirt, oil, dead cells, and all other impurities in the hair follicles. The most common sites where acne usually leaves problematic lesions or scars are the chest, neck, shoulder, face, and back. Lesions form due to acne and may resolve spontaneously, but in some individuals it may take a fairly troubling course. Nonetheless, with some effective treatments, as well as lifestyle and diet modifications, you can effectively manage your acne without much difficulty.

What causes acne?

Knowing the factors that contribute to acne is helpful in formulating strategies to prevent or resolve acne. The following are the primary factors:

1. Excess sebum production
2. Pores which got clogged due to dirt and dead skin cell debris
3. Formation of bacteria in sebaceous gland

Overproduction of sebum blocks the skin pores and forms a whitehead (under skin) and blackhead (over the skin that may be open). Blackheads are black in color not because of dirt, but due to air entrapment which causes a chemical reaction when it interacts with the oily debris present inside of skin. Bacteria and yeast present in the skin leads whiteheads to form, which are pimples that are red, inflamed and filled with pus.

Normally almost 75 to 85% of all teens face some degree of acne problems during puberty. It is a natural process that results due to changes occurring in the biochemical or hormonal environment of the human body. Most of the teens are self-conscious about their physical appearance and looks, and when they experience severe acne problems, it can become difficult for them to handle it emotionally.

Most teens experience an improvement in their acne after growing up. However, it has also been observed that acne in some people may persist (or even get worse) beyond adolescence. Additionally, in some people, acne problems occur in their adult life due to some hormonal changes.

Factors that may worsen your acne

The following factors can intensify an existing case of acne:

- **Hormones:** androgens and hormones increase in girls and boys during puberty, during which sebaceous glands become enlarged and produce more sebum. Hormonal changes associated with pregnancy and consuming oral contraceptives may also increase the production of sebum.
- **Certain medications:** drugs which contain lithium, androgens and corticosteroids promote acne.
- **Diet:** according to several studies, some dietary factors—such as foods which include dairy products and foods containing carbohydrates, like bagels, chips, and bread—raise blood sugar, which can also cause acne problems.

If you are experiencing acne, do not feel overwhelmed. Acne responds fairly well to diet and lifestyle modifications (such as limiting your sugar and dairy intake, maintaining personal and physical hygiene by bathing daily, and avoiding excessive sweating). If your acne does not resolve due to lifestyle modifications, you should seek expert help. There are several over-the-counter medications that also help in resolving acne.

Take away lessons:

Chronic health issues of any sort should not stop you from living your life; especially today when you have excellent medical and therapeutic options available to manage your illnesses.

Framework for Preventing Chronic Disease and Promoting Health

Life Span and Settings
- Worksites
- Schools
- Communities
- Health Systems
- Infants
- Children and Adolescents
- Adults and Older Adults

Priority Conditions
- Heart Disease
- Stroke
- Cancer
- Diabetes
- Obesity
- Arthritis
- Oral Health

Underlying Risk Factors
- Tobacco
- Nutrition
- Physical Activity
- Alcohol
- Genomics

The key to a healthy, disease-free life is to:

- Consume healthy nutrition (and you will learn more about it in subsequent chapters)
- Learn about stress-relieving techniques like meditation, regular exercise, and yoga
- Maintain healthy sleeping habits
- Keep up with your periodic medical examinations and follow your medical treatment plan religiously
- Incorporate healthy habits and avoid drugs, nicotine, and alcohol.

Parents, teachers, healthcare providers, and the government have a responsibility to help you live a healthy life.

It is important to keep in mind that the journey to a healthy life goes as long as you live.

Self- Assessment for Chapter 3

- *What are some common health issues that are usually reported in teens?*
- *Are you at risk of developing obesity; why or why not?*
- *How can you prevent chronic metabolic/medical illnesses?*
- *Why do teens develop acne at the time of puberty?*
- *Prepare an action plan to manage moderate acne without medications.*

CHAPTER 5
BUILDING RELATIONSHIPS

Getting old comes with responsibilities. There is a responsibility to be more independent (both in making relationships and maintaining healthy bonds). However, as easy as it may seem, sometimes building relationships could be quite challenging, which is why we will discuss some difficulties that you may encounter in making bonds and how to overcome these problems.

Highlights of this chapter

- *Communication*
- *Relationships*
- *LGBT*

COMMUNICATION – THE PILLAR OF STRONG RELATIONSHIPS

The Four Communication Skills

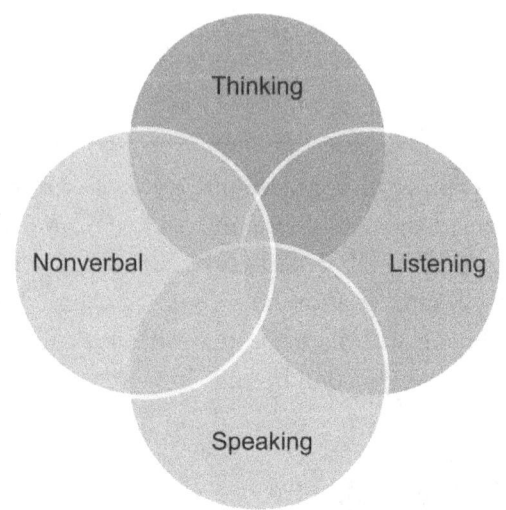

You met Carey in Chapter 1

Carey was the active, smart and complete package cheerleader who was excellent at everything she does. Just like a typical teen, Carey was very fond of making new friends and living a fun-filled life (her motto was work hard and play harder).

She met John at a friend's party and they both fell for each other. The first couple of weeks were like magic. However, as time passed, Carey realized that John was quite different from what she initially thought.

He was pretty casual, and never took the initiative to call or plan to meet. At times he often felt very distant. Sometimes she felt that it was only her who was blabbering and John was not even listening carefully. It frustrated her, annoyed her and stressed her out too...

She didn't understand if his growing lack of concern was because of any other relationship or because he was simply careless and insensitive.

Hours of worry, uncertainty, and stress started taking a toll on Carey's health and school performance. Once a super-achiever, Carey was just an average student after meeting John, and didn't feel like talking to anyone now. She waited expectantly for John to call, but he hardly ever called her.

It could have continued for weeks or maybe months until Carey decided to break it off. She said to herself—"I can't take it anymore. If he doesn't care for me, I shouldn't destroy myself for him either."

She called John and felt excitement and joy on the other side of the line. She asked if he wanted to see her this Friday and surprisingly he sounded excited and happy.

Carey didn't pay much attention. On Friday they met, but she was confused by his different demeanor. Carey couldn't stop sharing her grief that things didn't work out between them. She blamed John for not being so sensitive and caring as she had thought and seen other boyfriends were.

Before she kept going, she was surprised when John held her hand and told her how much he liked her and care for her. He told her how desperately he wanted to invite her to a friend's party when he called her the last time and how he stopped himself because Carey had an exam the same week.

He told her, "The only reason why I backed off is because I didn't wanted to pressure you to spend more time with me—you have a busy busy schedule. I mean that's what you always talk about..."

And Carey with her wide tearful eyes just said, "I wish we would have just talked instead of assuming things about each other."

Most of the times, when we are in a relationship, we assume things, like my partner is not paying attention to me because he is cheating on me; or I shouldn't ask him to go out with me because he is busy or something.

Why not just keep everything open?

Here are some keys to maintain good communication skills:

- Share your feelings at intervals (instead of keeping it locked in your heart). This applies to happy feelings as well as stuff that is bothering you.
- Be open and understanding. Try to take criticism in a positive manner.
- Be loving, caring, and respectful to other's opinions.
- Spend time with your partner and maintain healthy conversations.

FAMILY RELATIONSHIPS

Miscommunications and bad air are not limited to boyfriends and girlfriends only. Oftentimes, we have so much we'd like to say to our parents, like

- I want you to spend more time with me
- Or I want to go on a vacation with you

The same is true for parents who feel bothered or agitated at times because of your bad grades or because you are not giving them time or maybe because they don't like your friends (remember Adan from our Introduction, who is mad at his parents and his parents are mad at him).

Things become much easier when discussed and this rule is applicable to all relationships.

How to build a relationship with your parents

I have two news reports to share. I am sure you may have come across these (since they both stir national and international opinion).

The first story is of Rachel Canning

Rachel Canning sued her parents; however, the case was dismissed by the court.

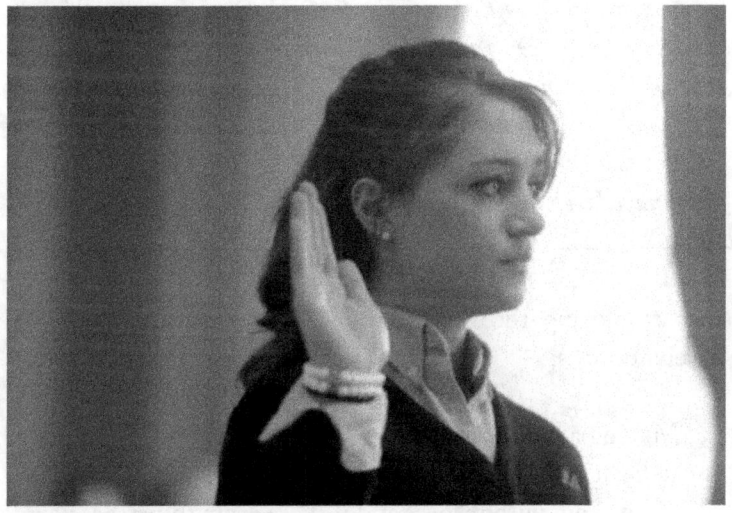

Rachel (a teen from Lakewood, NJ) has serious issues with her parents.

In a heated confrontation that stirred national and international opinions, Rachel accused her parents of being excessively controlling and abusive. She explained that they always bashed her regarding her weight and had issues with her boyfriend. After the confrontation, she claimed they kicked her out.

Sean and Elizabeth Canning (parents of Rachael) explained to the media and news that Rachel refused to follow the rules set by them (Rachel broke curfew repeatedly, a few times for alleged drunken partying). Rachel was also accused of stealing their money and bullying her sibling. They also said she ran away, first to her boyfriend's house and therefore emancipated herself from their guardianship.

Sean and Elizabeth Canning also said that Rachel could return home if she was willing to follow their rules. Rachel's parents both work full-time and also earn in the top 3 percentile of families nationwide.

Rachel told the court that her parents also promised her that they will be paying for her college education and she had always operated under this idea while growing up.

As part of the differences she had with her parents, Rachel's parents advised her in the fall of her senior year of high school that they were no longer providing her financial support. Rachel then sought legal help; her case didn't get any legal help (although it did evoke the disturbance, highlighting the uncontrolled and unmanaged teen-parent issues).

Besides employing the principles listed above, you can also work positively towards:

- Making a habit of spending some time together (even if it has to be at dinner table)
- Treat them with respect and if there is anything that you don't like or disagree with, feel free to discuss it with them
- Engage yourself in domestic chores (helping parents with grocery shopping, cleaning, or even just taking care of your own stuff)
- Express your love and care (even if you get little response in the beginning, it doesn't matter). Very soon your parents will get used to your attention and care and will return the same.
- Take initiatives in planning outings or events together as a family, like going to movies, picnics, or dinners.
- Share what is happening in your life and ask them how they are doing at work/ home

There are many advantages of maintaining a strong bond with parents and family as a whole. Not only will they have your back in bad times, but you can also look up to them for support, guidance, and love.

Research suggests that teens who have strong relationship with their parents are less likely to get involved in trouble.

BUILDING HEALTHY FRIENDSHIPS

Friends are a great help, not just in keeping us entertained, but also to guide us, support us, and stop us from making wrong decisions. We all make friends; but choosing healthy friendships is more important than having many acquaintances.

Although it may seem that making friends is easy, it sure is very difficult to maintain long-term healthy friendships that are free from:

- Peer pressure
- Violence
- Hatred/ grudges
- Unnecessary influence

Healthy friendships are those that bring out the best in you.

What are the principles of building healthy relationships?

The golden principles of establishing and maintaining relationships are the same (regardless of age, gender, or type of relationship).

These are:

1. Solving the problem/issue/conflict: One of the main discrepancies in today's relationships is avoiding the situation. Unless or until you decide to confront or face the problem, there is little chance of any improvement in the quality of relationships.

2. Taking care of each other regardless of the temporary conflicts or issues.
3. Giving and taking positive feedback. In any relationship, feedback is very important, not just for the bonding reasons but also for both the personality building of both the parties.
4. Effective and efficient confrontation
5. No holding grudges
6. Building trust and understanding
7. Asking and providing clarifications
8. Speaking only after thorough thinking (most of the times when we just say stuff, we end up offending or hurting other people).
9. One of the most important pillars of communication is listening. Make sure to listen to people around you (take their feedback, comments, and even constructive criticism). If you want to be a good communicator, you have to first become a good listener.

Activity

Think of a situation where good communication skills may have resulted in a different outcome

(Hint: It could be any relationship, school, friends, or neighborhood)

SEXUAL ORIENTATION – LGBT (LESBIAN, GAY, BISEXUAL, AND TRANSGENDER)

Before we discuss sexual orientation and activities in detail, let me share a few real life news reports that may effectively highlight the intensity of this problem and potential consequences of poorly handled cases.

Sexual orientation is your own choice and in some cases it is unintentional. Yet the problems or consequences that may follow should be handled appropriately (and not emotionally).

A 14-year-old Essex bullied gay boy fatally overdosed on prescription drugs

On 14 March at Colchester, Ayden Keenan-Olsen was found dead in his room by his father. The teen boy left two suicide notes that outline the gay racism and bullying he had experienced.

Ayden bypassed the security protocols on the home computer to research the practical methods to commit suicide by looking at methods on different websites.

Shy Keenan (Ayden's mother) who is also an anti-bullying campaigner explained at the hearing in Chelmsford that Ayden was assaulted and bullied several times for being gay at Colchester's Philip Morant school.

Robert James, the acting head teacher, gave evidence to defend the school's policies to deal with bullying. Mr. James said, *"As a school, our first priority is to make sure our students are safe."*

He also indicated that Ayden reported bullying on around 10 to 20 occasions since 2010 when school was started. The mother, Ms. Keenan, said that Ayden attempted suicide before (in October 2012) after overdosing on prescription pills.

Her son was a target of abuse, violence, and malicious allegations because of his Japanese ethnicity and because people believed he was gay, said Ayden's mother while crying bitterly during her evidence. Shortly before Christmas, he told his family that he was gay. Ms. Keenan stated: *"He said he was gay and had found somebody he thought he loved, but it was not reciprocated. We didn't care, we just loved him whatever. After Christmas it was like talking to a different boy – since he was able to say out loud to people that he was gay."*

Ayden was described as a sensitive child who wanted to plan his own anti-bullying campaign. He was a keen musician and idolized the television presenter Gok Wan. *"People would call him Gok as a compliment,"* she said. *"He tried very hard to look like him."*

Inspired from http://www.pinknews.co.uk/2013/11/15/uk-bullied-gay-teen-committed-suicide -by-overdosing-on-prescription-drugs -stored-at-school/

Well-defined and well-delineated gender identity is needed in order to maintain social, personal, physical and sexual relations with people of like mind and identity. As opposed to the traditional belief of just two genders—male or female—you may have often come across transgenders (people who underwent surgeries to transform into other genders).

In the similar fashion, most of us are heterosexual (have sexual interest in opposite genders, such as males are usually interested in females and females are generally interested in males when it comes to sexual relations), however, there are many people who are interested in the same sex (also known as homosexuals).

But here is the real deal:

- Is it normal to be a homosexual?
- Is it something to be ashamed of, or hide?

The simple answer is that choosing a sexual orientation or gender is your choice and personal business.

However, in some areas of the world, things work differently. In most Western countries, besides heterosexual males and females, other sexual varieties like transgender, gay, and lesbians are also accepted by law. However, it has also been observed that individuals who chose to be gay, lesbian or transgender are often discriminated against and rejected by society. They are also more at risk of being a victim of violence and discrimination.

Statistics and data on the LGBT population

You may be aware that the overall prevalence of the LGBT population is rising in almost all parts of the world (even in areas where religion has a very strong hold, suggesting it is something that is not in voluntary or political control). Statisticians and scientists have conducted meaningful research and surveys to identify the characteristics of LGBT population.

According to the latest estimates, it has been suggested that approximately 3.5% of the American population is gay, lesbian, or bisexual. This suggests a total of about 9 million adults (and this includes people who are openly gay or lesbians). When surveys were conducted to assess the population of transgender, a slight difficulty was encountered. Although, 0.3% (or 700,000) adults openly reported being transgender, it has also been observed that a lot of transgender individuals report themselves as either male, female, gay, or lesbian and that makes estimation quite difficult.

A few interesting facts about LGBT are:

- More people are transgender when compared to the combined of gay and lesbian population (1.8% vs. 1.7%)
- A lot of individuals have same sex encounters (about 8.2% or 19 million American adults report at least one such incident during their lifetime.

- More females tends to be bisexual than males

What may happen if you are gay, lesbian, or transgender?

According to statistics, it has been observed that homosexuals are at a greater risk of physical and mental assault by peers and society. Moreover, medical and mental illnesses, along with unhealthy behaviors, are also more common in homosexual teens (this includes tobacco, drugs and alcohol abuse).

Reports indicate that more transgender individuals are unemployed (despite having excellent credentials) and experience a higher rate of poverty, mainly attributed to social discrimination.

Other complications or side effects include:

Risk of attempting and committing suicide is 2-3 times higher in LGBT population due to psychosocial, medical, economical, psychological issues and social pressure as compared to non-LGBT population. Teens are at an even higher risk. Other social issues faced by the LGBT population are:

- LGBT population is a more frequently the target of homicide and violence. They often fall victim to discrimination and injustice.
- According to a national transgender discrimination survey, about 20% of all transgender individuals are homeless (20%). A lot of LGBT individuals face a lot of issues while looking for housing or residence options.
- The pay or salary scale of transgender population is often different from non-transgender (about 27% earns 20,000 or less per year)

Besides society and monetary issues, the LGBT population also suffers from sexual and/or verbal harassment, inappropriate inquiries about their sexual orientation, denial of promotions, and are forced to work in unfavorable working conditions. In most parts of the world, this subset of the population receives little to no help in terms of legal matters regarding retirement, employment, marriage, and adoption agencies.

Health Issues:

- High risk of physical damage to the anus and rectum
- Frequent visits to their primary care provider, and higher cost for medical bills due to perforation of the rectal wall, hemorrhoids, rectal tears, and bleeding episodes of rectum or anal fissures, ulcers and wounds, etc.
- Higher risk of developing, harboring, and transmitting sexually transmitted infections such as hepatitis, HIV, herpes, and anal cancer due to persistent trauma or inflammation in the rectal area.

They can also experience emotional trauma and psychological issues due to multiple break-ups and unstable relationships. This is also attributed to a lack of practical laws that allow marriage or other stable relationships in LGBT partners. An overall effect is:

- Multiple lifetime sex partners
- Higher propensity to get involved in unprotected, chance sexual and anal encounters.

Likewise, access to annual or periodic healthcare examinations to highly at-risk youth as well as the elderly LGBT population is also low due to social barriers and isolation. Other health related issues faced by the LGBT population include issues in getting health insurance and in most remote areas; even healthcare providers are not trained to identify and manage LGBT issues.

Another bullied gay teen commits suicide

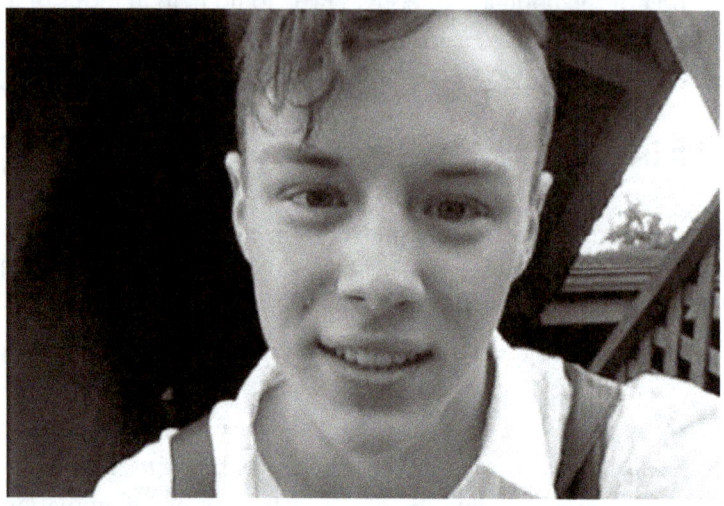

A 15-year-old teen boy, Jadin Bell, who was also a high-school sophomore in La Grande, Oregon has apparently killed himself by hanging after being bullied by his friends due to his gender preferences. He was put on life support after the hanging, but doctors and his family decided to terminate the life support, as no improvement was expected in his situation. The suicide was attempted in the playground of Central Elementary School. His family was told that he was bullied for being gay.

The news reported that this is the tenth suicide in the past 2 months and since the activist activities are so much on the rise, the pressure is also rising on the gay and lesbian population. Despite the fact that most parents and families are being more supportive to the teens who are homosexuals, peer pressure and bullying is rising.

The help is often delayed for such unfortunate teens, but this practice should be stopped!

Oftentimes, it has been observed that young teens who adopt homosexuality are rejected by their parents and families. There are many teens who face rejection, abuse, disrespect, and humiliation from families, but is there a solution?

Yes, in fact there are many. In almost all parts of the world, there are LGBT support organizations that provide political, physical, and monetary support to gay, lesbian, and bisexual teenagers.

Here is an example of the recommended behavior and approach that should be used by teenagers. Do not harm yourself or others. Instead report those people who are negatively affecting your life.

French Bus Driver Fired for Spraying Lesbian Couple With Water

Government and officials are now being more supportive and broad-minded for the LGBT population. This particular incident took place in France where a French public bus driver was fired from his job of driving after he sprayed water on a lesbian teen couple (who kissed each other good-bye before getting on the bus) according to news reports.

According to reports, the driver stopped the bus in front of a high school to pick up students around 5:30 p.m. on March 21. One of the female students kissed her girlfriend before boarding the bus. The kissing gesture apparently upset the driver, who showed his retaliation by allegedly removing the cap off a water bottle and dumping it over the couple. Moreover, when the teen asked the driver to stop at her destination, he told her to get off his bus and that he is "against homosexuality."

However, instead of getting into any fight or showing any type of response to the driver, the teens reported the driver. The French government took immediate notice of the complaint and the bus driver was fired because of his hateful speech and undesired behavior.

The transport service commented:

"The act cannot be tolerated and that's why the driver involved was immediately laid off as a protective measure."

http://www.edgeonthenet.com/news/international/News/156984/french_bus_driver_fired_for_spraying_lesbian_couple_with_water

How can you improve the quality of your life if you are an LGBT teen?

Sexual orientation and gender identity should not affect the quality of life of an individual, and efforts should be taken at an individual as well as a collective level to stop bullying or harassment of the LGBT population.

If you are experiencing bullying, sexual and/or verbal harassment, or any other type of social or peer pressure, do not give up. Standup for your rights and take your own stand. Include family and friends in the decision making process and seek help from organizations or third parties if you are under pressure.

Always remember that taking your life or inflicting harm to yourself because some ignorant people have an issue with it is not a sensible decision. Here are some tips:

- Perform physical activity and keep yourself fit
- If you are experiencing trouble, report it immediately
- Get counseling if you think the pressure is affecting your emotional or physical health.
- Avoid risky behavior in maintaining relationships
- Meditate regularly to minimize stress and stress-related complications.
- Keep up with regular and periodic healthcare examinations

If you have LGBT friends, relatives, or loved-ones, support them and love them instead of disrespecting or humiliating them.

Self-Assessment for Chapter 5

- How can you develop great communication skills?
- On a scale of 1 to 10, how will you rate your social and communication skills?
- What are some of the issues that are faced by the LGBT population?
- Are you aware of any potential victims of bullying or violence? How can you offer help or support?
- What may happen if optimal support and care is not provided to LGBT teens?

CHAPTER 6
TEEN SOCIAL MEDIA RELATIONSHIPS AND PRIVACY

This chapter is especially constructed to make you more aware of the potential hazards of social media sites (by sharing news stories). It is however, very important to maintain a safe and healthy social media presence.

This chapter discusses some essential and healthy tips that may provide help and necessary guidance to you.

Highlights of this chapter:

- *Sharing personal information*
- *Developing good social media relationship*
- *Posting pictures*
- *Having a healthy social media presence and why it's important.*

These days, it is very common to share information on social media sites. There are many sites that are designed in such a way that they encourage information sharing and network expansion. It is seen that teenagers fully embrace this public approach of social media and do not take steps in restricting their profile information. It is important to manage the privacy settings on social media.

- According to a survey done in 2012, teenagers like to share their personal information more now as compared to the survey done in 2006
- The popularity of Twitter among teens has increased significantly. It is observed that 24 percent of teens use Twitter, as opposed to previous prevalence of 16 percent in 2011.
- Most teens are Facebook users (with over 300 friends) or a minimum of 79 followers on Twitter.

A group discussion with teen shows their declining interest in Facebook, as they do not like the adult presence and lack of privacy, but beside all these issues they like to use the social media platform for socializing.

Hazards of Excessive Social Media Networks

Apparently, social media networks are great, but unsupervised and excessive use is hazardous. Here is why:

- More people start depending on virtual relationships and give less time and value to family and friends. This affects the social skills and ability to communicate with people effectively.
- Teens are often more likely to get obsessed with social media networks and spend most of their time taking and posting LOTS of pictures, sharing information, commenting and other activities). This not only takes a lot of time, but also affects productivity and quality of life.

SHARING PERSONAL INFORMATION

- According to a survey, 60% of teen users of Facebook like to keep their profiles private and most of the users manage their accounts with a high confidence level.
- It is observed that only 24% of teen users delete unknown people from their network or manage their accounts and mass information appropriately.
- According to a survey 9 percent of users show concern related to a third party accessing their data.
- Increasing network growth on Facebook gives the network variety in managing personal information and sharing information.

Teen committed suicide after cyberbullying incident

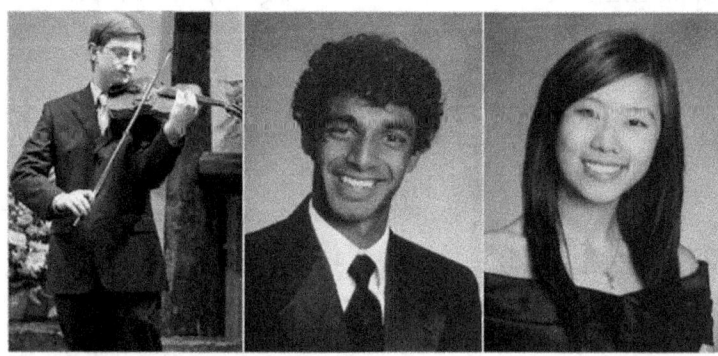

"Roommate asked for the room till midnight. I went into Molly's room and turned on my webcam. I saw him making out with a dude. Yay."

The authorities said that Mr. Ravi, a student of Rutgers University who was behind this message, used a camera in his dormitory room to allegedly stream the entire encounter of his roommate's intimacy live on the Internet.

Tyler Clementi, the 18-year-old freshman and an accomplished violinist, jumped from the George Washington Bridge into the Hudson River in an apparent suicide, just 3 days after being bullied by his peers due to his roommate's surreptitious broadcast.

Those who knew Mr. Clementi — on the Rutgers campus in Piscataway, N.J., at his North Jersey high school, and in a community orchestra — were anguished by the circumstances surrounding his death, describing him as an intensely devoted musician who was sweet and shy.

"It's really awful, especially in New York and in the 21st century," said Arkady Leytush, artistic director of the Ridgewood Symphony Orchestra, where Mr. Clementi played since his freshman year in high school. "It's so painful. He was very friendly and had very good potential."

The student who was behind initiating this campaign, Mr. Ravi, has been charged with two counts of criminal activities against a fellow student and is now awaiting trial. The other student, Molly Wei, whose room was used for recording and visualizing the private activities of the teen, has also been charged with two counts of breaching privacy. The prosecutor said that the maximum punishment of this type of assault is 5 years.

Chairman of the gay rights group Garden State Equality, Steven Goldstein, said the death of the teen is a hate crime that should be stopped. He further said that the community feels sick that the students are bullying their fellows by making surreptitious videos and are potentially destroying the lives of other people.

Inspired from: http://www.nytimes.com/2010/09/30/nyregion/30suicide.html?pagewanted=all&_r=0

HAVING A HEALTHY SOCIAL MEDIA PRESENCE

Teens like to share their positive experiences rather than sharing negative ones. Fifty-two percent of teens reported their online experience makes them feels good. A trend these days which makes teens crazy is sharing their personal information and current status update over their desired platform.

According to the latest statistics:

- It is observed that 91% of teen users post their photo, which was 79% in 2006
- In addition, 92% shared their real name in profiles
- 84% of teens shared their interests, like favorite book, music or movies
- 82% of teens shared their birth date, 62% shared their current relationship status
- 24% of teens shared their videos

What are the benefits of maintaining healthy social media relationships?

Healthy social media relationships are required to boost your confidence, networking skills, communication skills, and horizon. Social media networks allow you to meet new and very different and distinct people who you can explore and be friends with or without risking your safety or without having to actually meet them.

Perceived Effect of Social Networking on Social and Emotional Well-Being

Among the 75% of 13 to 17-year-olds with a social networking profile, percent who say social networking makes them feel more or less:		
	More	Less
Confidence	20%	4%
Depressed	5%	10%
Outgoing	28%	5%
Popular	19%	4%
Shy	3%	29%
Sympathetic to others	19%	7%
Better about themselves	15%	4%

http://www.huffingtonpost.com/larry-magid/kids-social-media-study_b_1629167.html

You can also seek help, assistance, and guidance from other people regarding assignments, studies or virtually anything. Even if you can get a good chat or good laugh by talking to someone, it is worth it.

However, there are certain limitations too. Oftentimes, teens get so obsessed with technology that it starts affecting their normal behavior and perception.

- 71% of teen users post their school name, which was previously only 49%
- 71% of teen users post their city, which was previously 61%
- 53% of teen users post their email address, which was previously 29%
- 20% of teen users shared their cell phone number, up from 2%

So a lot of numbers, but as you can see from the previous story, using social media irresponsibly can have devastating effects.

Below are a few real life stories that made it to the national and international news. Some ended tragically while other stories gave amusement and a good laugh to others.

The question is, would you let social media affect your life, family, career, and future?

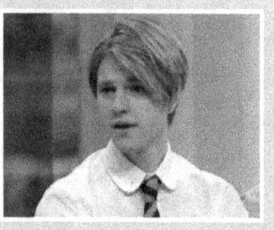

Seven members or associates of an East Bay gang have been indicted by a federal grand jury on charges that they took part in a spree of armed robberies of Safeway, Walmart and Rite Aid stores and boasted about their crimes on social media, authorities said Thursday.

Members of the Landry Crew bragged about their crimes on Facebook, Twitter, Instagram and YouTube, taking "trophy" pictures of themselves "literally rolling around in large amounts of cash and stolen items," federal prosecutors said.

Suicidal attempt by Danny Bowman

A teenager became so obsessed with taking the perfect selfie that he tried to kill himself when his efforts failed. Danny Bowman, 19, would spend 10 hours a day taking up to 200 photos of himself on his iPhone.

The teenager dropped out of school, remained housebound for six months and lost two stone in an attempt to capture the perfect self-portrait. Danny eventually became so depressed that he took an overdose, but he was discovered by his mother Penny and rushed to hospital.

He said "I was constantly in search of taking the perfect selfie and when I realised I couldn't I wanted to die. I lost my friends, my education, my health and almost my life."

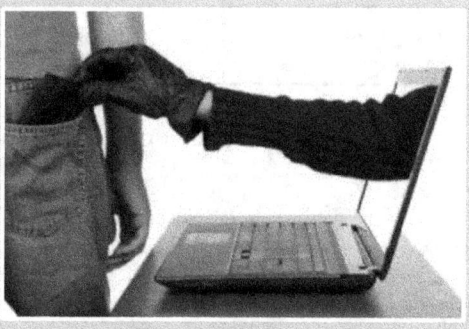

Teen boy raped 8- year old sister

A 13-year old British boy told police he raped his eight-year old sister because of pornography he saw on his friend's Xbox.

The teen, from Blackburn, England, pleaded guilty in court to indecently assaulting his sister and inciting her to perform a sexual act on him, the Lancashire Telegraph reports. He told police he had seen porn on Xbox and wanted to "try it out," and selected his sister because she was younger and "couldn't remember stuff."

MAINTAINING HEALTHY SOCIAL MEDIA RELATIONSHIPS

Danny, the obsessed teen who survived the suicide attempt sends a message to teens:

"People don't realise when they post a picture of themselves on Facebook or Twitter it can so quickly spiral out of control. It becomes a mission to get approval and it can destroy anyone. It's a real problem like drugs, alcohol or gambling. I don't want anyone to go through what I've been through."

Geisinger Health System pediatric psychologist Nicole Quinlan said:

"With social media, teens can literally be connected to all of these people 24 hours per day ... throughout the day or night. That leads to more positive contacts but also the inability to escape these negative or stressful things"

"People are putting their best face forward. If teens are making comparisons to others, they're doing so in what's really not a real-world setting and that can lead you to feel bad about yourself."

She also said that teens face academic pressure as well:

"There's also this expectation now that teens have the ability to get online and do all this extra research and they're expected to be able to access (assignments) at any time. They're constantly thinking about it ... Parents also have access down to assignment details, which in some ways is a good thing, but for some teens that adds an entire level of stress."

Moderation, Quinlan said, is the key to combatting social media stress.

Lindie Barnhart-Lloyd another teen said in an interview:

"You only get stressed if you allow yourself to be consumed with it. If you can't eat dinner with your family, watch an entire movie with your kids or take a walk without checking your phone, then you have a problem. Technology can be a convenience, but you can't let it be your life or then it's just another burden."

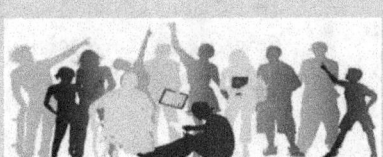

Some tips for you

- It is important to realize and prioritize your primary goals in life such as your academic and extracurricular performance at school and/ or work.
- Take an active effort at maintaining contact with real people around you (for your personal development and for the sake of productive relationships).
- Keep an eye on your overall consumption of social media networking and see if it is affecting your quality of life or preventing you from achieving your goals.
- Ideally, maintain a diary or notebook to keep a track of your goals is more helpful.
- Do not let social media sites distract you from your studies or normal daily activities, like sleep or naps (this can be accomplished by removing the apps from your cell phones and tablets).
- From time to time, take technology breaks and note your feelings about being unplugged.
- Always be very cautious while approaching and making new friends on social media forums. You never know who is behind a pretty face on the other side of the computer.

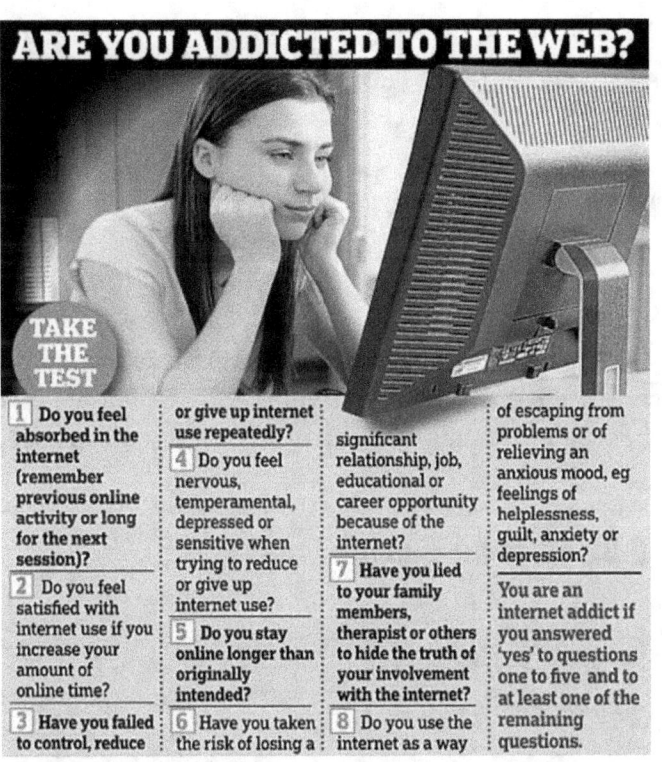

http://www.dailymail.co.uk/sciencetech/article-2015196/Too-internet-use-damage-teenagers-brains.html

Self-Assessment of Chapter 6

- How safe and secure is your social media network?
- How much time do you spend on social media sites per day?
- Is it difficult for you to complete other tasks because you are thinking about or on social media?
- Were you aware of potential hazards of social media sites?
- Are you in favor of maintaining privacy on social media forums? Why or why not?

CHAPTER 7
UNHEALTHY RELATIONSHIPS

How likely are you to fall in an unhealthy relationship? Most importantly, what are the signs of unhealthy relationships and how can you safely and soundly walk out of an unhealthy relationship safe?

Highlights of this chapter:

- *Dating Violence*
- *Bullying*
- *Peer Pressure*

15-year-old Sammy has always been in love with 17-year-old Michael, who was her childhood friend too. Everything was going great until Michael dropped out of high school and started doing drugs.

Things were tough for Sammy, and on top of that, Michael has violent mood swings and attitude issues. Sammy is now thinking of breaking up with him, but fears Michael's possible violent reaction.

- *Should she continue the relationship and wait for a good time to break up?*
- *Should she report her physical abuse to concerned authorities?*

Unhealthy relationships are a part of life, but somehow, teens are seemingly more involved and affected as a result of dysfunctional relationships.

How can it affect you?

Statistics suggests that dysfunctional teen relationships often take a toll on physical and emotional health. Involved teens often suffer the most and their personal and academic life is affected the most.

- Unhealthy relationships can lead to substance abuse issues, peer pressure, bullying and involvement in criminal activities.
- The risk of sexually transmitted infections, unwanted teen pregnancy, miscarriage and other reproductive or gynecological issues also increases.
- Most unhealthy or dysfunctional relationships end in chaos if steps are not taken in a timely manner. This may even include death of either partner due to suicide or homicide.

Case of a missing teen.

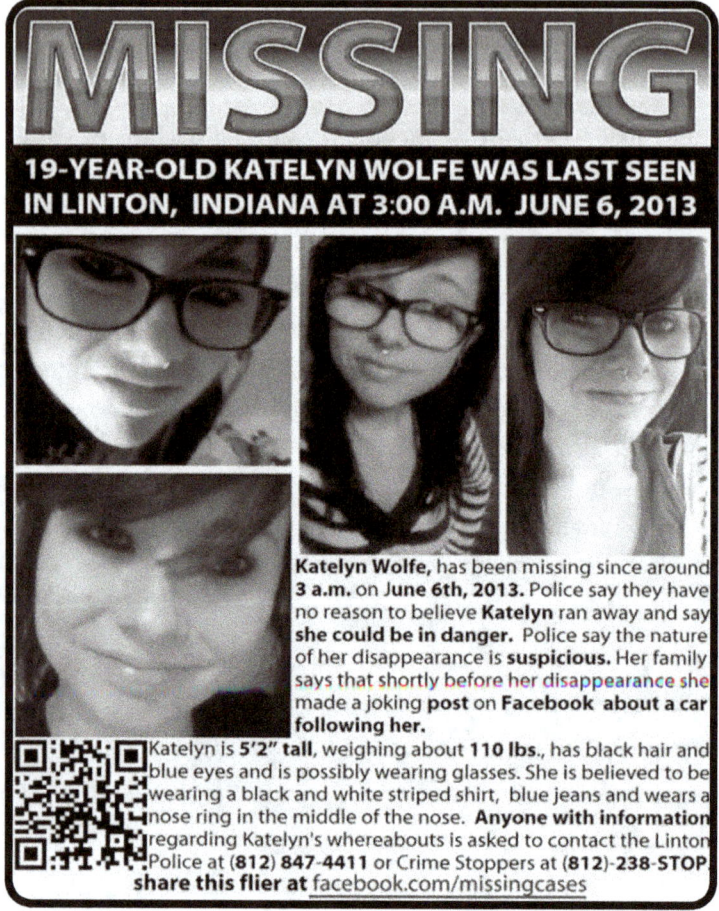

Unfortunately a few days later, I came across this news update

19-year-old Linton woman died from asphyxiation, body found in water

The Linton Police Department announced late Monday that state conservation officers located a body around 5 p.m. believed to be a missing 19-year-old Linton girl.

According to an advisory issued by the police department, the identity of the body has not been confirmed, but there is enough information to lead officials to believe the body is that of Katelyn Wolfe. Authorities said the body was discovered in a rural area in Sullivan County. The exact location is not being a rural area in Sullivan County. The exact location is not being disclosed at this time. Police do suspect foul play in Wolfe's disappearance and are treating the death as a homicide.

Linton Police Chief Troy Jerrell announced late Monday that two people were in custody in connection with Wolfe's disappearance. Randal E. Crosley and Jordan W. Buskirk are preliminarily charged with murder.

Wolfe, 19, has been allegedly killed within hours of being kidnapped.

Police said Wolfe knew at least one of the two men in custody.

http://fox59.com/2013/06/11/body-found-in-greene-county-possibly-katelyn-wolfe/#axzz2a6Qz5b4m

Dating Violence **10 WARNING SIGNS OF ABUSE**	
• Checks your cell phone or email without your permission	• Makes false accusations
• Constantly puts you down	• Mood swings
• Extreme jealousy or insecurity	• Physically hurts you in any way
• Explosive temper	• Possessive
• Isolating you from your family or friends	• Tells you what to do

SOURCE: Love is respect

What can you do about it?

- Education and learning is the key. If you think you are in an unhealthy relationship, do not wait for a bad event to happen. Gauge the risk by assessing the warning signs and take timely interventions.
- Seek help; if you are suffering or has suffered emotionally, counseling is fairly helpful. For more serious risks, speak to a responsible and trustworthy adult.
- Develop excellent communication skills to manage issues and sort out solutions.

DATING VIOLENCE

DATING AND TECHNOLOGY

Digital tools - social media, text messaging, and emails - have given bullies and abusers a new way to control, degrade, and frighten their victims anywhere, at any time, even when they're apart.		
1 in 4 dating teens say they are abused or harassed online through texts by their partners	**2X** as many teenage girls than boys reported sexual abuse online and through texts	**LESS THAN 1 in 10** victims of digital dating abuse sought help

SOURCE: *URBAN Institute Sept. 2013*

Tristan Stahley, a 16-year-old Pennsylvania boy, was arrested Saturday night after allegedly stabbing his 17-year-old girlfriend to death in a park, CBS Philly reports.

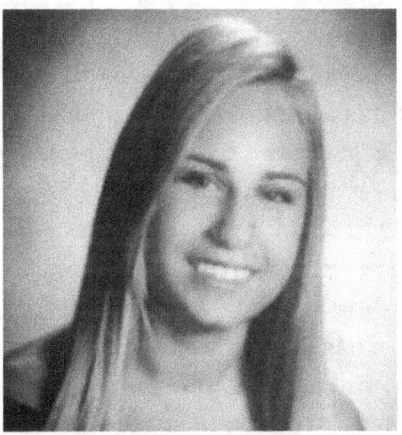

A teenage girl is dead after her boyfriend stabbed the teen along a suburban Philadelphia hiking trail. Pennsylvania State Police say Julianne Siller, 17, was killed Saturday night by her 16-year-old boyfriend Tristan Stahley during a break-up.

The teens left the Stahley's Skippack Township, Pa. home around 8:30 p.m. and headed for Palmer Park along Creamery Road in Skippack Township, Montgomery County, Pa. Skippack is about 30 miles northwest of Philadelphia.

Investigators say the couple was walking along a nearby trail when they got into an argument over Siller "going out too much." Siller then smashed Stahley's cell phone, according to state police. Then Stahley allegedly pulled out an orange-colored folding knife and stabbed his girlfriend in the throat and body.

Stahley told police he then dragged her body off the trail and into the woods to conceal the murder.

Police say the teen then went home. His mother, Heather Stahley, told investigators it appeared Tristan had been crying and that he had blood and dirt on his legs.

When Heather asked her son what was wrong, he wouldn't explain, saying he would tell her if the two went for a walk. Police say the two then left the house for a nearby trail and during the walk Tristan confessed to the crime. Heather asked her son if he was joking and after he replied "no" he began hysterically crying, according to the criminal complaint.

The teen explained the couple was breaking up when he stabbed Siller. Tristan told his mother he was going to kill himself because he couldn't go to jail. The mother and son then returned home at 9 p.m. where Heather alerted the authorities.

In the meantime, Tristan waited outside.

His father, Brian Stahley, told police that when he went outside, Tristan had another knife to his neck and told him to stay back. The father and son then got into a struggle as Brian tried to wrestle the knife away. He was eventually able to get the knife, but was scratched in the face and bitten on the hand, according to police.

BUT HERE IS WHAT YOU SHOULD KNOW

Investigators say the two dated for about nine months. Friends told NBC10's Daralene Jones that the couple had various issues, but Siller wanted to stick it out because she believed she could "fix" Stahley, who was a recovering drug addict and on medications for depression.

Stahley is being held without bail. He is charged with first-degree murder, third-degree murder and possession of a weapon.

http://www.nbcphiladelphia.com/news/local/Teen-Boy-Accused-of-Stabbing-Girlfriend-to-Death-on-Hiking-Trail-208985431.html

What should you do if you are in an abusive relationship?

If your partner abuses you, restricts you from meeting other friends or loved-ones, or keeps unnecessary tabs on you, it is important to realize that you ARE in an ABUSIVE relationship and it is very important for your mental, physical and emotional health that you get out of the relationship before it is too late.

Oftentimes, we don't want to give up like Julianne Siller, but is it really worth it?

It is also very important to break-up while also considering a safe and secure passage.

The following tips are of significant help to prevent chaos:

- Always try to call off the relationship by phone, text, or email instead of meeting the person at a secluded location
- If you are expecting a violent reaction, make sure to inform your parents or loved ones before making this decision
- If you feel threatened, do not hesitate to contact authorities and get a restraining order in case your ex starts stalking you.

BULLYING AND PEER PRESSURE

It doesn't matter if a person is old or young, rich or poor, experienced or naïve—they will always be influenced in one way or another by the people surrounding them. This influence is commonly referred to as "peer influence" or "peer pressure." This may be negative or positive, but either way it always affects the mindset, mood, habits, and ultimately the life of an individual.

Peer pressure and bullying —a direct relation?

To establish a relationship between bullying and peer pressure, you must understand fully what peer pressure is. It can be defined as the influence from our surroundings that impact our attitude, thoughts, daily practices, or the decisions of a group or an individual.

Therefore, if a child is teased for being fat, or a young girl is insulted in front of her class because she has braces, etc., other children around will also make fun of them. This may include teasing them directly, leaving nasty notes or targeting them on a social website. Other children might do this to feel a part of a social group, to gain acceptance, or just to protect themselves from being bullied.

Investigators say a Marion middle school student used a tie to hang herself Monday morning.

During a briefing Monday afternoon, investigators said 14-year-old Braylee Rice left gym class between 8:40 and 9 a.m., went out to the bleachers near the track and used the tie to hang herself. Police said no one saw the seventh grader kill herself, though students and a teacher found her at the bleachers. The coroner listed her time of death at 10:25 a.m.

The school said there had been speculation about bullying related to the student's death, but added that it was too early to know if that's the case. The school didn't dismiss for the day, although parents could pick their children up at their discretion. The school was never on lockdown, district officials said. Grief counselors were on hand to talk to students, and students and staff and will continue to be made available as needed.

http://fox59.com/2013/05/06/police-middle-school-student-used-tie-to-hang-herself/#axzz2xAv1qOd1

Why do kids do it?

One of the most obvious reasons why kids may find themselves pressured to bully another child is simply because they see this as the easiest way to fit in. Others may feel that bullying someone will get them respect in the eyes of their peers. And some may bully because this may ensure that they will not be bullied themselves.

Real story of Teen Bullying that ended in a tragedy

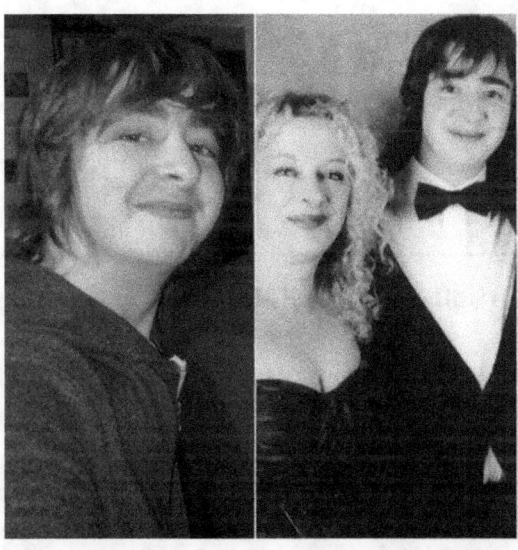

A schoolboy has killed himself after being falsely accused as a rapist by a gang of drug dealers who were reported by the kid.

Tom Acton, 16, gave information to officers about the gang selling the drugs near his residence.

A hate campaign was then begun by the gang of snarling thugs.

His mother Gaynor said they were like "a pack of wolves hounding a wounded animal."

They accused him of tying up and raping a girl. The mentally tortured teen began to self-harm and isolated himself.

Just a few days before he was set to appear in court to testify, the boy was found to be critically ill.

Three days later, he died in the hospital. The cause of the death is yet to be determined.

What should you do?

You must first realize that being the target of bulling is definitely not your fault, and it can be dealt with. It is also wrong, and you do not (and should not) tolerate it or allow it to happen to someone else. With proper guidance, your parents may be able to help you both avoid and prevent bullying altogether. Even though you may have a notion for independent decision-making and may try and handle it yourself, you shouldn't. Bulling is both dangerous and serious, and should be handled by an adult, and by someone who's in a position to deal with this issue before it gets out of hand or leads to a devastating outcome.

Self-Assessment for Chapter 7

- How can bullying or peer pressure affect your life?
- What should you do if you are experiencing bullying?
- How satisfied are you with your relationships?
- What are some signs of an abusive relationship?
- What should you do if you are in an abusive relationship?

CHAPTER 8
DEVELOPING CHARACTER

Highlights of this chapter:

- *Character and Trustworthiness*
- *Respect*
- *Responsibility*

"Character cannot be developed in ease and quiet. Only through experience of trial and suffering can the soul be strengthened, ambition inspired, and success achieved."

—Helen Keller

Some values, manners, and etiquettes are taught in school, but there are a number of things that you learn from interactions and personal dealings. For example, character building and trustworthiness, respect for others, and taking and sharing responsibilities are some characteristics that differentiate and delineate you from your peers.

Jack and Tim were childhood friends, mainly because their parents have been good friends and neighbors for the past 25 years. Seventeen-year-old Jack was good friends with Tim, despite having objections with some of his habits and values. The differences were bearable until last summer.

During their last summer vacation, when Jack and Tim were playing near a park, they found a wallet. While Jack wanted to return the wallet, Tim resisted and they ended up in a small quarrel. Although Tim was not convinced, Jack took the initiative and contacted Mr.

Frank, the gentleman to whom that wallet belonged (with the help of some business cards in the deeper pockets).

Needless to say, the man was very happy after receiving his wallet and he did offer some money as a reward, which Jack declined (once again it was against the wishes of Tim). But just within a couple of years, Tim also realized the power of maintaining good character and doing good deeds when he applied for an internship and Mr. Frank conducted his interview and later offered him the position.

Being a teen is often challenging, as there are so many temptations. You might steal, lie, do drugs, cheat on exams, and even engage in fun (but illegal) activities, but there are always consequences of evil things.

How can you be trustworthy and reliable?

Obviously, if you offer help, support, and care to others and build a strong character, people will trust you and respect you more.

Here are some pillars:

- Always be honest to yourself and to people around you. Truth always prevail no matter what and dishonest people are never trusted
- Never deceive, steal, or cheat (this applies especially to situations where your chances of being caught are negligible)
- Be reliable and dependable. Keep your promises and don't share secrets
- Have the guts, power, and courage to take right decisions at the right time (no matter how hard it is)
- Take serious efforts in maintaining a good reputation
- Support and love your family, friends, and loved-ones—no matter what
- Treat everyone fairly

A person of sound character always plays by the designated rules and sets rules and restrictions on his or herself. This means that it is not supposed to be all fun and no pain.

Walter Anderson said something that you should always remember:

"Bad things do happen; how I respond to them defines my character and the quality of my life. I can choose to sit in perpetual sadness, immobilized by the gravity of my loss, or I can choose to rise from the pain and treasure the most precious gift I have—life itself."

RESPECT

We all love people who are associated with us, but are we able to respect every person who is around us?

Every day we come across cheaters, frauds, those who don't keep their promises, and those who hurt others; some people lie for financial gain, while others do it just to support a habit…but what is the long-term impact of such nasty behaviors?

How can you earn the Respect of your peers and loved ones?

Respect is hard to achieve, as it is a deep-seated feeling. People will only respect you if they think you deserve being respected. Same goes for other people. If you show them respect, they will return the favor. It is hard to expect other people to love you and show concern for you when you don't respect them.

You will see many examples around you where teens disrespect their parents, teachers, or elders. What do you think about them?

Most importantly, how would you feel if someone behaved in the similar fashion toward you when you are old? (Definitely not good)

Here are some golden principles of giving and earning respect:

- Be accepting and tolerant of differences
- Always display good manners and etiquettes. It is not that hard, just treat the people in the same way you want them to treat you
- Avoid using bad language
- Always show empathy, compassion, and mercy toward others (even if you think that they don't deserve it)
- Try to be considerate of the emotions, sentiments, and feelings of other people
- If you have power, strength, or control, do not abuse it. Do not hit or threaten other people who cannot fight back
- Conflicts and differences exist—with parents, friends, peers, and other people in your surroundings. But the solution of disagreement is not to fight or quarrel. If you are confused or uncertain, seek help and clarification instead of working with incomplete or flawed knowledge

RESPONSIBILITY

Barbara and Sandra are sisters with a 3-year age difference between them, but despite being the younger of the two sisters, their parents depend more on the judgment and commitment of Sandra. Needless to say, Barbara always feels jealous and somewhat ignored by the gesture of her parents.

After fighting herself all these years, she finally had it when her parents gave Sandra the responsibility of distributing the invites for Barbara's birthday. Having feared that her friends were going to make fun of her, she retaliated, and finally took the responsibility of distributing the invites.

- Would she be successful?
- Is jealousy the only required motivator to achieve a goal?

I highly doubt it.

Responsibility comes from a number of things. You have to engrave it in your personality.

Most of you have come across similar situations, when your parents, teachers, friends, or other loved ones prefer someone when it comes to giving a task or responsibility.

In fact, when it comes to you, I am sure you have your own favorites or preferences (let me share, I always trusted my mother more with certain urgent tasks because despite all my love for father, I knew deep in my heart that he would forget, because of his busy schedule, or maybe wouldn't do the job as perfectly as my mother would).

- What makes you choose someone over somebody else?
- What could make someone choose or prefer you over another person?

The answer is simple….

What are the basic principles of responsibility?

- If you undertake a task or job, fulfill it no matter what. In case you cannot fulfill it, do not wait until the last moment. Instead of taking cover or hiding, face the person and tell them why you can't do a certain job. It is more important to earn the trust of the other person than to feed your false pride or ego.
- In order to fulfill your commitments, always plan ahead of time to minimize the risk of last minute delays.

Some tasks or jobs are easy to begin with, but when you start doing it, these may become challenging. What can you do at that time? Should you just abandon and walk away or should you try harder? (Definitely the second option)

You are all aware of Michael Jordan, the great legendary American basketball player.

He once said:

"If you're trying to achieve, there will be roadblocks. I've had them; everybody has had them. But obstacles don't have to stop you. If you run into a wall, don't turn around and give up. Figure out how to climb it, go through it, or work around it."

Here are some other principles that may help in incorporating the classic principles of responsibility in your life.

- Try to give your best shot at everything and never slack (no one respects or trusts slackers).
- There are temptations, so many distractions may lure you away from your task or assigned responsibility, but it is your self-control and self-discipline that can help you in achieving your goals.
- Making commitments, offering help, and taking the responsibility is very easy. Anyone can do that. If you want to be different and superior, try considering the consequences before taking the responsibility.
- If you took a responsibility and messed up, do not take cover or hide, accept the failure and take accountability. That's the only way you are going to learn.

Activity:

Here is an activity....

- Write the names of three people you love most, but are irresponsible
- Write the names of three people you think are very responsible, although they are not really close to your heart

Now close your eyes and think for a moment. If it comes to a critical decision, who would you listen to or believe? The one you love most or the one you trust most?

The same logic applies to other people as well. If you don't present yourself as the most trustworthy, reliable, honest, and responsible person, you are least likely to get any respect or recognition from other people.

How can you adopt responsibility, respect, and character traits?

Although it is believed that a lot of such traits are learned with time and with maturity, you can incorporate healthy habits early on by:

- Sharing responsibility of household stuff with your parents and siblings (like doing your laundry or dishes, or helping your mother with grocery shopping)
- Volunteering at school or after work (learn more ideas in the chapter on community services and volunteering)
- Joining summer camps (or other outdoor activities) where you can learn to contribute, share workloads, and fulfill responsibilities
- Save money and take care of your own expenses
- Get a part-time job to learn how to take accountability for your actions
- Try to help elderly family members in their tasks (such as shopping, reading, or with food)
- If you have younger siblings, it is a golden opportunity to offer them support, help, and guidance

How does adopting these traits help you in your future life?

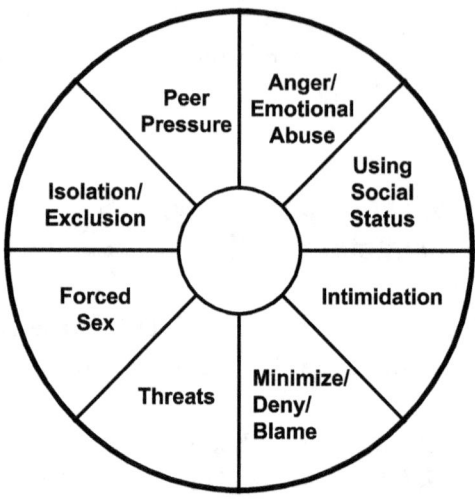

This is the question you must be thinking; why go through all the hassle, effort, and hard-work. Of course whatever we do, it is to ensure that somehow we will benefit in the future.

Here is how adopting these traits could help you in moving ahead:

- If you are responsible in making relationships, you are less likely to be a victim of dating violence, sexual abuse, or physical abuse (discussed in subsequent sections).
- If you are trustworthy and respectable, your peers and other associated people won't push or pressure you for illicit or undesired behaviors.
- If you have a strong character, you won't get in trouble for common teen issues like drugs, drunk driving, alcohol consumption, sexual violence, and other crimes.
- Having your own set of rules and being more responsible in maintaining relationships also reduces your chances of teenage

pregnancy, contracting sexually transmitted infections, and other such issues.

In fact, just recently a survey report was published by Microsoft, to which teens responded with great concern that if their online reputation is damaged (as a result of careless, reckless behavior online), they will have difficulty getting accepted to a good college (a sign that indicates teens are becoming more and more aware as well as responsible in their dealings).

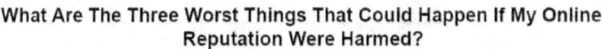

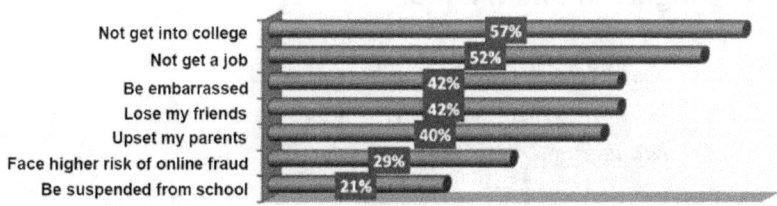

http://www.microsoft.com/security/resources/research.aspx

Assessment for teens

1. How can you improve your trustworthiness and responsibility?
2. What are the benefits of adopting these traits (other than those that are listed in text) and avoiding problems, such as teenage pregnancy, STDs, etc?

CHAPTER 9
YOUR MENTAL AND EMOTIONAL HEALTH

Highlights of this Chapter

- Your Mental and Emotional Health
- Understanding your emotions
- Managing stress
- Mental and Emotional Disorders
- Suicide
- Substance Abuse
- Alcohol, Tobacco, and Drug Use
- Community Service
- Meditation
- Success Principles

YOUR MENTAL AND EMOTIONAL HEALTH

EMOTIONAL
Coping effectively with life and creating satisfying relationships

ENVIRONMENTAL
Good health by occupying pleasant, stimulating environments that support well-being.

FINANCIAL
Satisfaction with current and future financial situations.

INTELLECTUAL
Recognizing creative abilities and finding ways to expand knowledge and skills.

WELLNESS

SOCIAL
Developing a sense of connection, belonging, and a well-developed support system.

PHYSICAL
Recognizing the need for physical activity, diet, sleep, and nutrition.

SPIRITUAL
Expanding our sense of purpose and meaning in life.

OCCUPATIONAL
Personal satisfaction and enrichment derived from one's work.

Oftentimes, your parents, teachers, and other elders stress the need of maintaining a healthy lifestyle in order to stabilize and strengthen your physical health. A recent survey also suggested that most teens are well aware of different strategies and tips to maintain their physical health, yet the concept of maintaining mental and emotional health is very unpopular.

Why is that so?

It is true that most adults believe that stress and stress-related issues are uncommon in teens or adolescents. Most adolescents ignore potential stressors and warning signs by not seeking any medical help for the management of emotional issues. But did you know:

- *The overall prevalence of depression, anxiety, and stress -related disorders in teens are as high as 5 to 70% (surprisingly, this rate is higher than even the adult population).*

- *Another report suggested that the lifetime prevalence is 20% in the teen population, as opposed to 12% in the adult population.*

What may cause stress?

Oh this is not a tough question, as you all have your stressors. Some adolescents are more focused on getting good grades at school, while others just want to be popular and likable in their peer circle.

Stress was once referred to as a relative term, yet over time, scientists and investigators have developed several theories, exams, and protocols to investigate stress and related risk factors that may lead to stress. Below is a list of the top ten risk factors that may lead to moderate to severe stress.

TEENAGE STRESS
THE TOP TEN*

1. School
2. Family/parents
3. Friends
4. Work
5. Sports
6. Homework
7. Lack of Sleep
   Love Life
8. College
9. Appearance
   Extracurricular activities
   Grades
   Relationships
   Tests
10. Lack of time

* **Note:** This list reflects multiple answers from a test group of ninety 10th grade students. The number 1 answer was listed by almost 50% of the students. The number 2 answer was listed by 30% of the students and the number 3 answer was included by almost 20% of the respondents.

How to manage stress?

There are different strategies that may help in managing and controlling stress levels. Each person has a different capacity to bear stress and manage their issues. Below are a few tips that may help in managing stress:

- Maintain a social life, as loners are at fairly high risk of developing stress -related disorders.
- Limit your intake of fast food or junk food, as nutrition has a very strong association with the secretion of certain hormones that may lead to stress.
- Maintain a balance between your personal, social, and school life.
- Identify your risk factors and instead of avoiding the situation, it is much better to face the problems.
- Avoid drugs, tobacco, alcohol, and other chemicals or harmful substances that may alter your health.
- If you think your stress levels are interfering with your day-to-day activities or impairing your quality of life, feel free to consult a therapist.

What happen if you don't manage your stress?

Medical issues—yes, when you get stressed out or worried, your body goes into a defensive mode and release a lot of stress hormones, such as cortisol. Going into a lot of details regarding cortisol is beyond the scope of this book (and probably a little too boring for you), so keeping it simple and short, you should know that excessive cortisol leads to acne, abnormal glucose levels, and weak bones.

Other long-term effects of high stress levels are:

- Poor activity or low physical activity that may lead to obesity. In most cases, depression is also coupled with eating disorders

- Depression and psychological issues that may lead to suicide, homicide, or other forms of self-harm or violence
- Poor self-esteem
- High risk of chronic medical issues like diabetes and hypertension
- Acne and pimples (which I have written about in detail in other chapters) but one of the most common causes of uncontrolled acne is high serum cortisol concentration
- Insulin insensitivity syndrome: cortisol increases blood sugar levels, thinking your body and brain needs a lot of energy to sort out issues, but if you take longer in looking for a solution, persistently high glucose levels can lead to insulin independent diabetes mellitus

MENTAL AND EMOTIONAL DISORDERS

Understanding your emotions:

- *It is normal to feel angry, sad, disappointed, or agitated when things don't go your way*
- *It is normal to feel happy, excited, or overwhelmed if anything good is happening (like meeting new people, making new friends, getting good grades on exams)*

But what should you do when you are very angry, sad, or upset?

When you are happy, how should you celebrate your success or happiness?

As an adolescent, it is important to understand that happiness or success shouldn't be celebrated with alcohol, tobacco, or drugs. And in case of any sad event, taking revenge upon the innocent people around you by violence is not going to help your situation or solve your problem.

What may lead to abnormal emotional behavior in teens?

It is believed that optimal emotional health is directly linked to the domestic environment and social circle of teens. Oftentimes, individuals who are less responsible surround teens. According to a report by renowned child psychiatrist Helen an inability to control mood and emotions is not only associated with a very high rate of high school drop-outs but is also directly linked to violence and involvement in crimes.

Several research scientists have identified risk factors that contribute to unhealthy emotional health. A few well-known triggers are:

- Unhealthy family environment (that may include history of aggression in parents)
- Living in a stressful surrounding (exposure to violent fights or high street crime)
- A known history of domestic violence, and/or substance abuse in parents

How can you manage abnormal emotions?

The human brain is extremely complex; you may develop all type of emotions. It is up to you to know what is good from what is evil. However, it is not necessary that you manage all the issues and problems by yourself. Here is what you can do:

- Seek help from your parents. Discuss and share what is bothering you and how they can help.
- It is understanable that we don't always want to share everything with our parents. We need space and we want to maintain our image. But there is always a trusted 3rd party in the form of a sibling, friend, or a relative.

- You can also seek help from a medical provider, your parent, school counselor, or teacher.
- Your family care physician is indeed the most reliable person to talk to (considering the fact that healthcare providers are obligated to maintain confidentiality).

SUBSTANCE ABUSE

Are you aware that?

- In the United States, approximately 30% of teens (or one in three teens) are exposed to at least one friend or close relative who abuse prescription drugs to get high
- More than 1.75 million American teens reportedly consume illicit drugs
- Half of the teenagers reported that they have thought about consuming prescription drugs at least once in the past 6 months
- Majority of teens believe that prescription drugs are safer than street drugs

Substance abuse eventually involves all the organs and the damage is more devastating because the brain and brain pathways in teens are in developmental stages. Intake of any chemical that affects the normal balance of brain chemicals can increase the risk of impaired brain development several folds.

What are the most commonly abused drugs amongst teens?

It is logical that somehow all the drugs that are abused by adults are also accessible to teens.

The most common ones are listed below:

Hallucinogens includes all popular street drugs; such as psilocybin, THC, LSD, mescaline, peyote DMT, PCP, and MTF

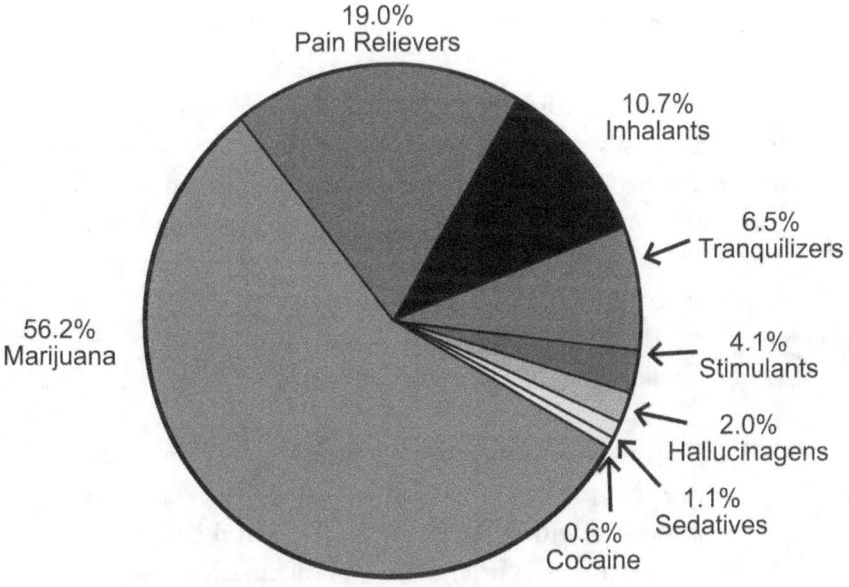

2.7 Million Initiates of Illicit Drugs

The current incidence of hallucinogen use in adolescents is as high as 2 – 6%. Ecstasy is used by more than 5% of the adolescent population for recreational use (especially in clubs) and is highly associated with abnormal and excessive sexual activity (that further contributes to the increasing rate of sexually transmitted diseases and teenage pregnancy).

Inhalants:

Several factors like easy availability, low risk potential, and cheaper cost makes this variety of illicit drugs as the most popular variety in teens; however, most teens have no idea how strong and disastrous this drug could be. Moderate intake of inhalational agents can lead to permanent damage to vital tissues like the nervous system, respiratory system and gastrointestinal tract. The most common varieties include solvents (like ether), butane, aerosols and glue.

Marijuana:

So far, the most common, most frequently consumed (and somewhat easily available) drug is marijuana. According to reported statistics, approximately 56.2% of the entire adolescent population consumes marijuana on a regular basis (and more than 85% reported that they have consumed marijuana on at least one occasion).

Other popular drugs used by teens are:

- Cocaine - with over 3 million teen users, it is indeed one of the most disastrous drugs and has been associated with a large variety of physical and mental complications. A brief overview is discussed in the table below.

Cocaine affects every system in the body and can lead to: Heart attack, abnormal heart rhythms, elevated blood pressure, fluid in the lungs, decreased blood flow to the heart, kidneys, testicles, and intestines. It can also cause seizures, headaches, blood clots, and bleeding in the brain.

With approximately 2.6% of the teen population consuming cocaine, it is a huge economic and productivity loss.

- Painkiller or analgesic abuse is also becoming extremely common (with an estimated 10-fold increase over the past 5 years. Popular analgesic agents with high abuse potential are opioids and tramadol.
- Other drugs include sedatives (4.8%), Ritalin (2.3%), Oxycodone (3.6%), Salvia (3.4%) tranquilizers (4.6%) and other cough medications comprise 5.0% of the entire pool of illicit drug abuse.
- Drugs that directly affect the brain (either acting as a stimulant or as a depressant by interfering with the normal brain secretion of hormones or chemical mediators) are also becoming extremely common. Most frequently used agents are benzodiazepines, Cannabinoids, amphetamine and Methamphetamine, alcohol, and Barbiturates.

How teens get their hands on these drugs?

Is that a secret?

Most teens get their first exposure to drugs from friends or family members. Here is a chart that reflects how teens develop addiction or dependence.

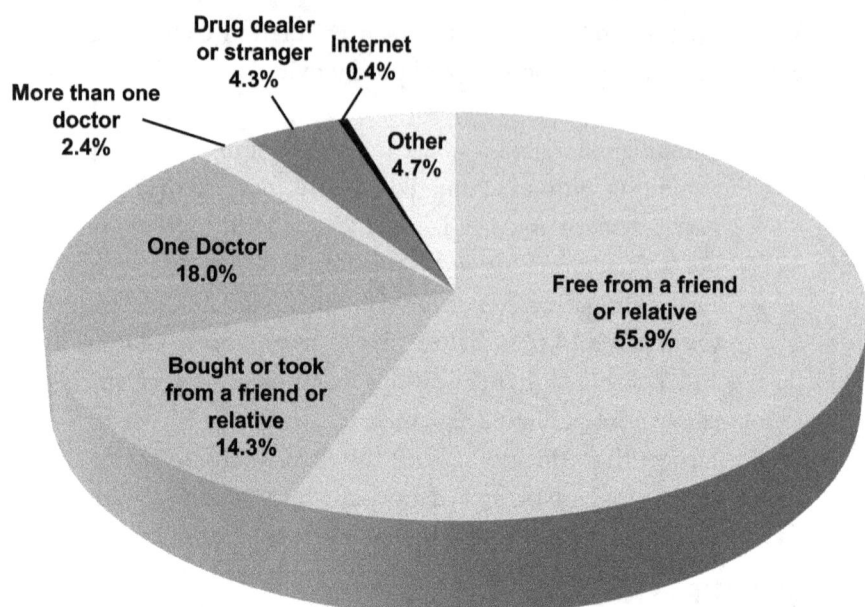

Who is at risk of developing drug abuse?

Risk factors that promote drug abuse in teens	What factors help in managing drug abuse problem?
Abnormal home environment (domestic violence or history of parental drug abuse) Loners, socially isolated teens Personal or family history of mental illness Stressful lifestyle (troubled academia, low motivation, poor aspirations and goals for future)	Excellent upbringing Positive family bonding and support from friends and loved ones Excellent aftercare Strong motivation Support groups

History of sexual abuse at a younger age Depression Ineffective parenting Peer pressure	

What are the hazards of drug abuse in teens?

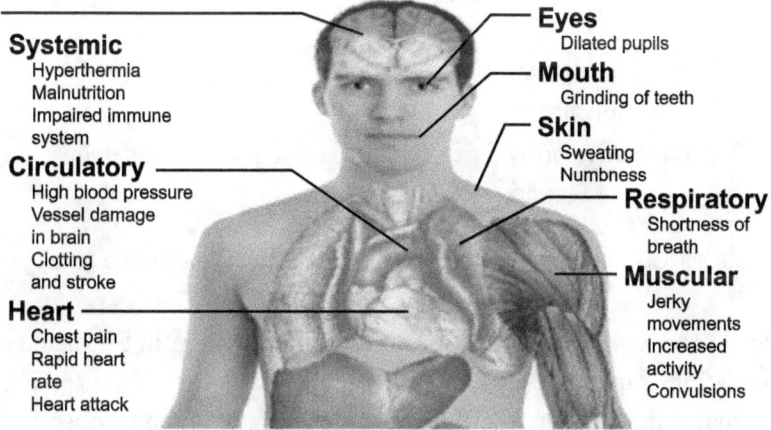

- Teens who abuse drugs have a higher risk of death due to drug overdose.
- Teens who abuse drugs for a longer period of time eventually develop multi-organ dysfunction that may increase morbidity and permanently compromise the quality of life.
- Young female teens who develop drug dependency are at a higher risk of becoming teen moms.
- The risk of developing sexually transmitted infections is very high in teens who abuse drugs than in the general population.
- Diseases like gonorrhea, Chlamydia, syphilis, herpes and HIV are the common sexually transmitted infections/diseases.

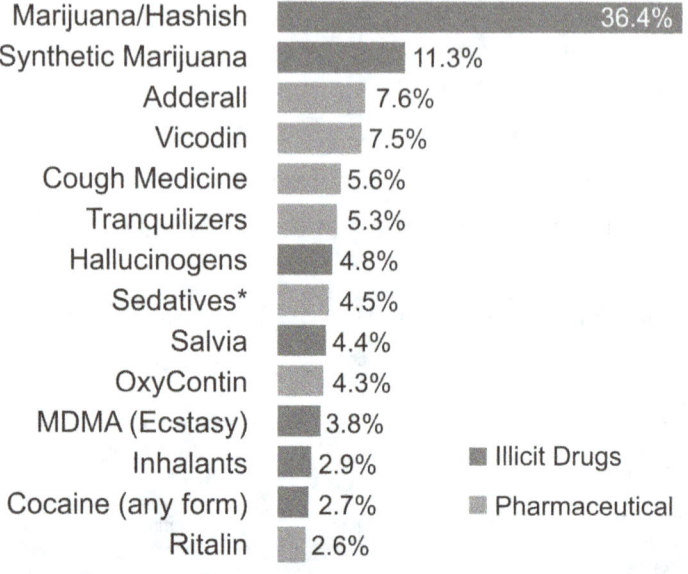

SOURCE: University of Michigan, 2012 Monitoring the Future Study

The list above shows the most commonly abused drugs in the teenage population. The report also suggests the increasing trend and spiking rate that is indeed a matter of huge concern. It is commonly observed that apart from the availability of drugs, certain other factors that largely account for the intake of drugs are:

- Peer pressure (or social influence of friends who consume drugs).
- Ineffective parenting or a history of drug abuse in the family.

TOBACCO USE

It has been observed that over the years, smoking and tobacco use is increasing in adolescents at an alarming rate. Most adolescents take up smoking as a trend or just to impress their peers, yet unknowingly, they develop dependence and then addiction.

Are you aware that:

- Statistics suggested that 90% of smokers take up smoking before the age of 18.
- Records from Centers for Disease Control (CDC) suggested that more than 5.6 million adolescents are expected to die at a younger age due to complications of long-term cigarette smoking.
- CDC data also indicated that more than 3,200 adolescents (under the age of 18) take up smoking each day in the United States.
- Data from 2012 suggested that roughly one-quarter of all high school students are current tobacco consumers.
- Most common tobacco products that are used by adolescents are: cigarettes, cigars, smokeless tobacco, hookahs, pipes, snus, kreteks, bidis, and dissolvable tobacco; whereas the use of flavored cigarettes and electronic cigarettes is more popular in younger adolescents.

What causes addiction in cigarette smoking?

Cigarette smoking or tobacco use in any other form (chewing tobacco) is equally bad and harmful to health in the short term as well as the long term. The addictive component in tobacco is nicotine, which is the main habit forming element.

Research suggests that most adolescents take up smoking just to get peer acceptance and approval, others develop this habit due to pressure and stress (that may be domestic, personal, or academic).

Other risk factors that increase the risk of tobacco consumption in adolescents are:

- History of smoking in family (especially smoker parents). Besides environmental influence, a positive family history of smoking increases the sensitivity and genetic attractiveness to tobacco and nicotine

- Adolescents from low socio-economic families
- Impulsive or violent personality
- History of trouble at home or school
- A relative or absolute lack of parental guidance and support

Increasing use of Hookah in adolescent population and the negative impact of inadequate knowledge:

In lieu of all the diseases and disorders that are associated with smoking, governments and non-government organizations have initiated a number of public awareness campaigns. The good thing that came out of this negative publicity is a slight decrease in the overall prevalence of tobacco consumption by teenagers, *but is it really true?*

Indeed not; a recent study has suggested that more teens now consume tobacco in other forms such as hookah, e-cigarettes, and other varieties like shisha. Teens believe that the hazardous effects of tobacco are minimal with hookah consumption as compared to cigarettes because:

- Hookahs utilize water vapors as a medium to channel the flavor that reduce the toxicity
- The long tube decreases the amount of total tobacco consumed

But the fact is that hookah is even more hazardous because unlike cigarettes, there is no filter to stop the large particles of toxins from getting in your system. Consequently, all the health hazards are at least 1.5 times more severe in regular hookah users.

What are the disadvantages of tobacco use in teens?

Research and data has proved that cigarette smoke contains over 300 carcinogens (carcinogen is any substance that is capable of causing cancer with prolonged exposure). Long-term smoking increases the risk of cancer involving the stomach, esophagus, colon, anal region, cervix, urinary bladder, lungs and other organs.

- Long-term cigarette smoking is associated with chronic respiratory difficulty marked by health issues like asthma, chronic obstructive pulmonary disease and other ailments
- The risk of inflammatory and infectious diseases increase in adolescents who consume tobacco on a regular basis.

Management of nicotine addiction:

Are you aware that once you develop nicotine dependence, going back is not easy?

Just as there are programs to manage alcohol addiction and drug addiction, some hospitals and centers also offer treatment for nicotine addiction. Chain smokers should start off by tapering their nicotine consumption by using nicotine gums (that decreases the desire to smoke by delivering small quantities of nicotine in blood), or nicotine patches (which serve the same purpose and are often used for managing tobacco dependence).

It is important to discourage teens from consuming tobacco as most child psychologists call smoking a gateway to more hazardous forms of addiction, such as heroin, marijuana, and cocaine. Government and communities should also take serious efforts to minimize tobacco use in adolescents by:

- Imposing higher tax rates on cigarettes
- Passing laws that would prevent teens from buying cigarettes
- Creating public awareness and proper guidelines regarding the effects of cigarette smoking on an individual's health

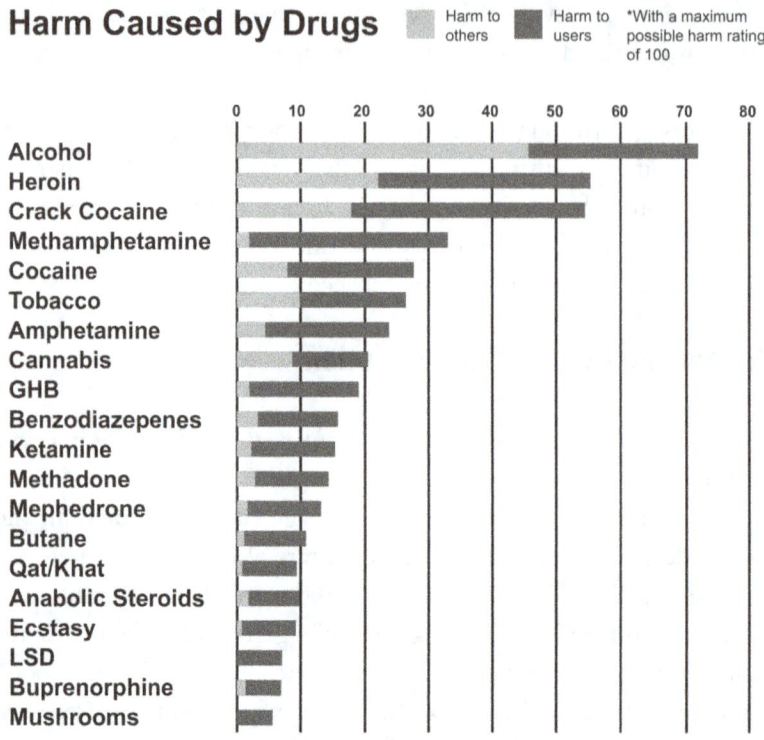

Adapted from "Drug harms in the UK: a multi-criteria decision analysis", by David Nutt, Leslie King and Lawrence Phillips, on behalf of the Independent Scientific Committee on Drugs. The Lancet.

But here is what you should see—it has been reported that a drug-dependent individual is a threat to society and to himself. Here's how:

- A drug-dependent teen is more likely to evolve into a drug-dependent adult (who can be a burden to his/her family and society).
- Drug dependent individuals are more likely to get involved in risky behaviors (such as driving under the influence, engaging in the casual sexual encounters, carrying and transmitting sexually transmitted diseases, and become pregnant teens).
- Drug users are more likely to engage in acts of violence, crimes, and abuse than a non-user. The cause is mainly impaired

judgment, clouding of consciousness, unnecessary rage, and agitation.

Here is a real life story that depicts how drugs like meth can impair judgment and leads to irrational behavior in teens, sometimes as hateful as murder.

Pregnant 17-year-old who 'was high on meth when she murdered cop as he tried to help her' faces court

- *Megan Grunwald is facing more than a dozen charges for a fatal car chase last month*
- *Sheriff's deputy Cory Wride approached Grunwald and her boyfriend on the side of the road because he thought they were having car trouble*
- *The murder set off an hours long car chase which ended in officers fatally shooting Garcia-Juaregui*
- *In her first court appearance Monday, her lawyers said she is 'scared to death' of facing life in prison*
- *While sitting in his squad car, 27-year-old boyfriend Jose Angel Garcia-Juaregui opened up the rear window and shot Wride dead*
- *Grunwald is now being charged with Wride's first-degree murder and several other felonies as an adult*

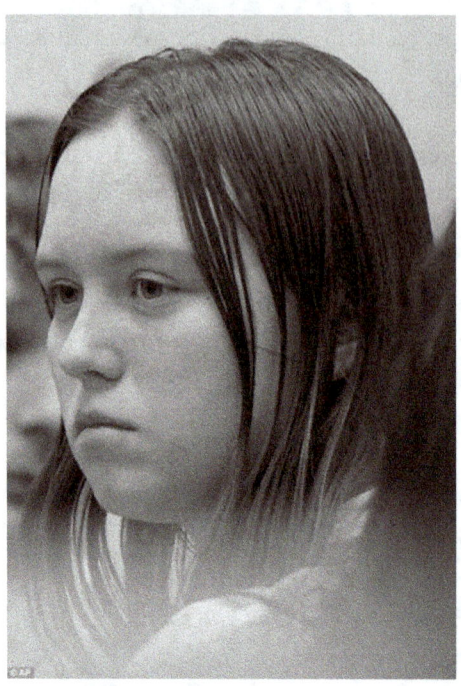

The 17-year-old girl charged with the January shooting spree that killed one police officer and wounded another made her first appearance in court on Monday, with her lawyers saying she is 'scared to death' of facing a maximum sentence of life in prison.

Looking solemn and dressed in a yellow jail jumpsuit, Meagan Dakota Grunwald, of Draper, appeared in front of a judge in Provo, Utah, to face accusations she was high on meth when she and her boyfriend shot and killed a sheriff's deputy who was trying to help them with car trouble last month.

Grunwald, who is being held at the Salt Lake County jail, is charged as an adult with aggravated murder, a first-degree felony, and 13 other charges related to the January 30 events.

She is accused of driving her pickup truck while her boyfriend allegedly shot and killed one police officer and wounded another, the *Salt Lake Tribune* reported.

Life in prison without parole is the maximum penalty the teen could face if convicted of aggravated murder.

http://www.dailymail.co.uk/news/article-2567240/Pregnant-17-year-old-murdered-beloved-cop-road-boyfriend-high-meth-scared-death-facing-life-prison.html

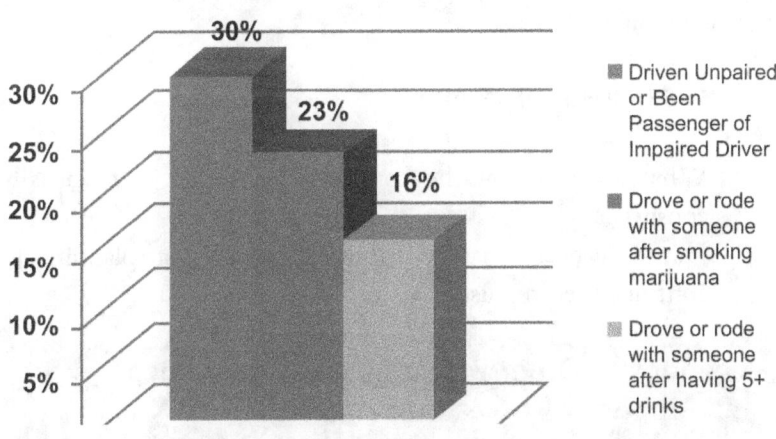

What should you do if you develop drug dependency?

The realization that drugs are not for recreation is indeed the first step, but how do you get to this first step?

It is pretty simple; just answer a few questions and you will know if you should continue drug abuse or not?

- You may get a temporary sense of high soon after consuming drugs, but how long does your euphoria last?
- Do you get headaches, body aches, nausea, vomiting, shivering, feverish or feelings of being sick if you don't consume drugs for a considerable period of time?

- Life is short, so are you enjoying the love and care of your loved ones to the fullest?
- Are you hopeful for your future?
- Do you think you will be able to continue this dependence on drugs for months or years and still be able to compete with your friends and peers?
- Most importantly, would you like your kids to consume drugs?

If your answer to most of these questions is negative, you should consider adopting practical strategies to quit drugs, and/or seek professional help.

Self-Assessment for teens:

- What are some of the common drugs that teens usually consume?
- Have you ever consumed drugs? If so, are you planning to continue the drug use?

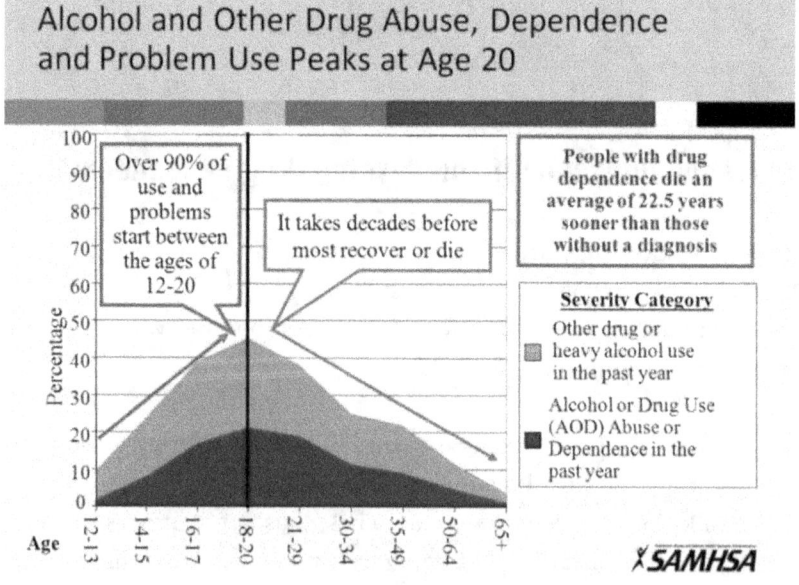

ALCOHOL ABUSE

I have a real news story to share (it is sad because the teen was charged quite recently).

News Story: Connor Hanifin

A teenager who was critically injured in a crash earlier this year that killed his friend has now been charged with vehicular homicide.

Ocean County prosecutors say 18-year-old Connor Hanifin of Toms River turned himself into police there on Monday. He was later released after posting his $75,000 cash bail.

The charge stems from a Feb. 8 crash in Toms River that caused the death of 19-year-old Toms River resident Francis Duddy.

Prosecutors say it appears that Hanifin was speeding when he lost control of his car and struck a tree. They also say alcoholic beverage containers were found in the vehicle, and testing showed Hanifin's blood-alcohol level exceeded the legal limit.

http://www.oceancountysignal.com/2014/03/24/toms-river-teen-charged-with-passengers-death-in-fatal-crash/

Although, alcohol consumption is illegal under the age of 21 years in most parts of United States, approximately 70 to 85% of teens have reportedly consumed alcohol (at least once) before their 18th birthday.

If you or your peers are consuming alcohol (or thinking about consuming alcohol) by utilizing secret means, you should know that it is a crime.

But when your parents, teachers, or loved ones stop you from consuming alcohol, it is mostly for other reasons. Alcoholic teens are more likely to get involved in criminal and violent activities, and in some circumstances may even die as a result of it. Driving under the influence not only threatens the life of the driver, but the passengers, pedestrians, and other drivers as well.

A small reckless behavior and an hour of enjoyment can compromise your entire life, destroy your career, and may put you behind bars for the rest of your life.

UNDERAGE DRINKING STATS

Nearly 1/3 of all drunk driving deaths happen to people ages 16-20.

1/3 drunk driving deaths: 16-20 YEAR OLDS

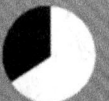

There are about 10.8 million underage drinkers in the United States.

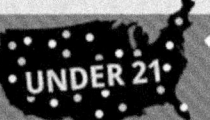

One in six teens binge drinks.

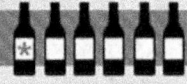

Only 1 in 100 parents believes his or her teen binge drinks.

100 PARENTS

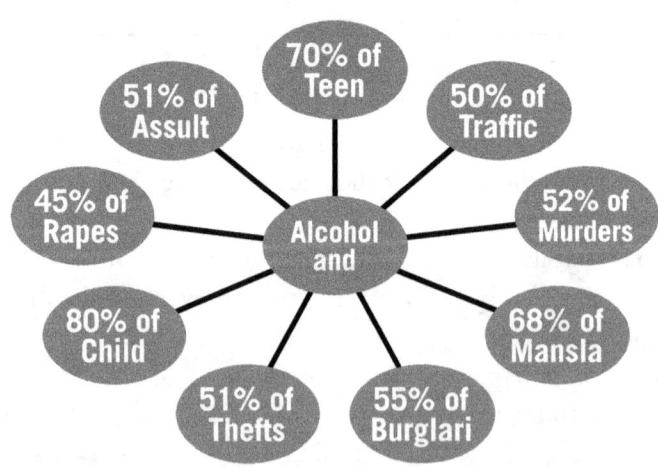

Alcohol and
- 70% of Teen
- 51% of Assult
- 50% of Traffic
- 45% of Rapes
- 52% of Murders
- 80% of Child
- 68% of Mansla
- 51% of Thefts
- 55% of Burglari

The prime reason for all of the above is impaired judgment due to alcohol consumption. In addition to accidents and assault, drunken teens are more likely to commit moral crimes like sexual assault or physical assault. Moreover, alcohol intake often leads to other drugs and intoxicants that further affect your health, career, family life, and potential of a bright future. But is that all?

Moderate to high alcohol intake can deteriorate your health and may lead to multi-organ damage. As you may know, alcohol is metabolized by the liver; unfortunately, consumption of excessive alcohol (with or without other irritants) can lead to compromised liver functioning. If left untreated, alcohol consumption can slowly lead to liver cirrhosis, liver failure, and eventually death.

It is also important to realize that the liver is not the only organ affected; prolonged alcohol consumption affects neurological functioning, dietary intake and causes damage to the heart. Since alcohol contains a lot of irritants that agitate the lining of the stomach and gut, the risk of ulcer related conditions is also very high.

Below is a brief summary of the potential systemic complications of alcohol intake in teens and adults.

The Long Term Health Effects Of Alcohol

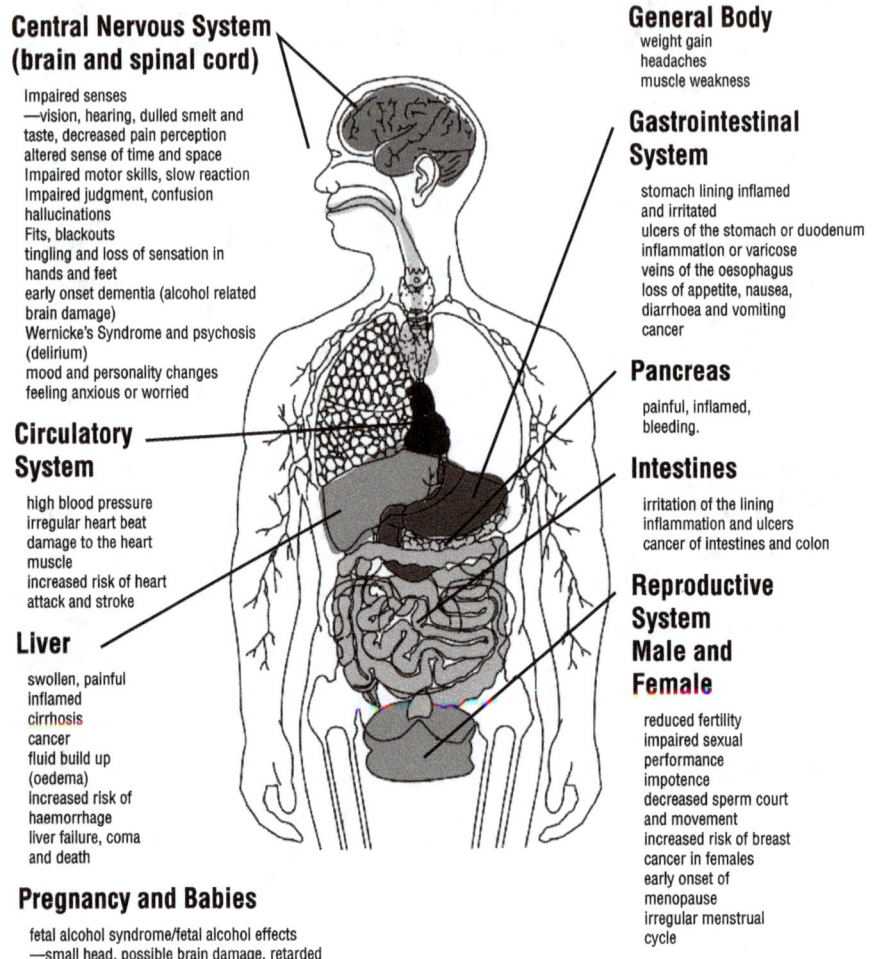

Central Nervous System (brain and spinal cord)

Impaired senses
—vision, hearing, dulled smell and taste, decreased pain perception
altered sense of time and space
Impaired motor skills, slow reaction
Impaired judgment, confusion
hallucinations
Fits, blackouts
tingling and loss of sensation in hands and feet
early onset dementia (alcohol related brain damage)
Wernicke's Syndrome and psychosis (delirium)
mood and personality changes
feeling anxious or worried

Circulatory System

high blood pressure
irregular heart beat
damage to the heart muscle
increased risk of heart attack and stroke

Liver

swollen, painful
inflamed
cirrhosis
cancer
fluid build up (oedema)
increased risk of haemorrhage
liver failure, coma and death

Pregnancy and Babies

fetal alcohol syndrome/fetal alcohol effects
—small head, possible brain damage, retarded growth and development

General Body

weight gain
headaches
muscle weakness

Gastrointestinal System

stomach lining inflamed and irritated
ulcers of the stomach or duodenum
inflammation or varicose veins of the oesophagus
loss of appetite, nausea, diarrhoea and vomiting
cancer

Pancreas

painful, inflamed, bleeding.

Intestines

irritation of the lining
inflammation and ulcers
cancer of intestines and colon

Reproductive System Male and Female

reduced fertility
impaired sexual performance
impotence
decreased sperm court and movement
increased risk of breast cancer in females
early onset of menopause
irregular menstrual cycle

Alcohol and drunk driving:

Of course, besides harming the body, alcohol, as we just read, also impairs judgment. Teens who drive under the influence are more likely to drive recklessly and thus often become victims of traffic accidents.

Besides the high mortality, DUI is also associated with permanent disability and a huge economic burden on the families for:

- Handling of court cases to minimize sentencing
- Payment for reconstructive surgeries
- Payment of damages to those impacted by the drunk driving of the teen

Drugged driving on the rise

Recorded crashes involving drugs are up 22 percent since 2006, even as those involving alcohol-only have dropped 25 percent

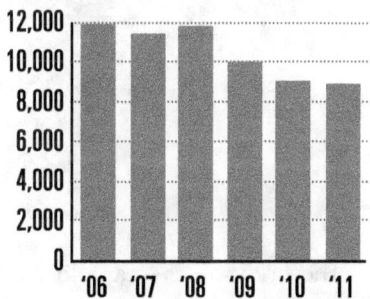

Alcohol-involved crashes

Drug- and alcohol-involved crashes

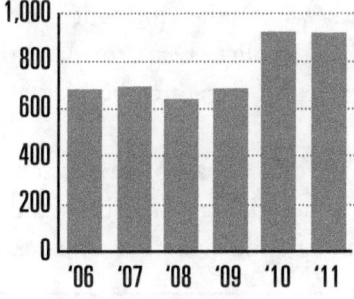

Drug-involved crashes

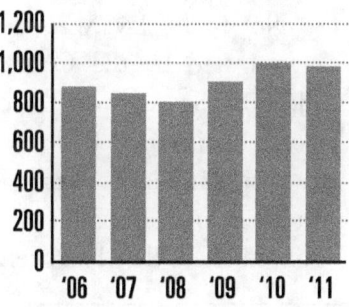

SOURCE: Michigan State Police drunken-driving audits

Alcohol poisoning:

Teen's Death Linked to Alcohol Poisoning

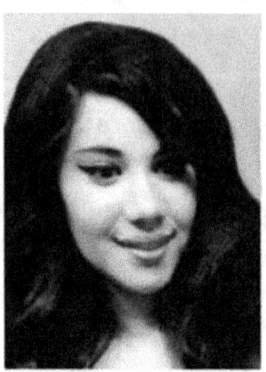

The body of 15-year-old Mireya Mata-Alvarez was found in the backseat of a car according to the authorities. Forensic reports suggested that she died of alcohol poisoning.

No foul play was detected when the incident was investigated by the Council Bluffs Police Department. In addition the Autopsy/Toxicology report suggested accidental alcohol poisoning.

A preliminary investigation revealed that Mata-Alvarez had been out all night with two other girls and five boys and police believe they had been drinking and smoking marijuana.

Indeed, most of you are already aware that alcohol (if consumed in large amounts) can lead to alcohol poisoning, a term that denotes loss of blood pressure control, loss of consciousness, weakening of pulse, severe nausea, vomiting, diarrhea, coma, and ultimately death.

Possible risk factors for alcohol poisoning include binge drinking (consumption of large amounts of alcohol after short intervals of time). Binge drinking acutely increases the blood alcohol concentration (since liver cells can only lower alcohol levels at a fixed rate).

Alcohol exerts its actions by acting as a central nervous system (CNS) depressant and thus leads to coma and a delirious state; here are a few signs of alcohol poisoning.

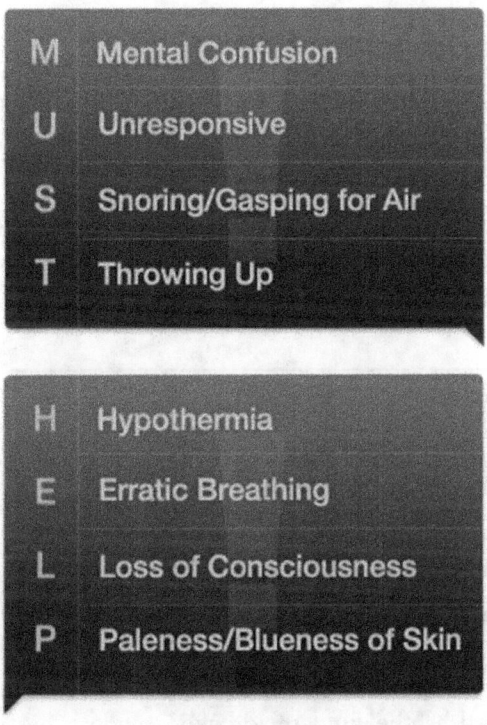

M	Mental Confusion
U	Unresponsive
S	Snoring/Gasping for Air
T	Throwing Up

H	Hypothermia
E	Erratic Breathing
L	Loss of Consciousness
P	Paleness/Blueness of Skin

Self-Assessment for Alcohol intoxication

1. What are the hazards of alcohol poisoning in teenagers?
2. How can alcohol affect your health in the short term and long term?
3. Why shouldn't you consume alcohol at a younger age? Explain briefly the legal and economic complications?

TEEN SUICIDE

A young person usually attempts to end his/her life in utter desperation or frustration only. However, any act of carelessness and hopelessness eventually devastates the whole family, community, and friends. Every person wonders if they could have done things that may have kept that person from committing suicide. It is important for teens to understand why and how teens actually attempt or commit suicide and how they can help themselves and others avoid such a devastating event.

Here are a few real life stories that stirred despair and pain for the community and Blake's loved ones.

The mother of a Westfield teen who took his own life last week is speaking out, hoping to save lives in his memory.

Blake Boothe, 14, passed away on March 12.

"Everybody just loved him. They just loved him," Blake's mother, Heather Boothe, said.

Blake was artistic, had a unique point of view and is being remembered as the kind of kid who made a big impact on his friends. Last week, though, the unthinkable happened. Heather said **Blake's suicide came after he was picked on – even bullied – in part because he was openly gay.**

"*I honestly don't think that he wanted to commit suicide. I think it was just a split second decision,*" Boothe said. If it wasn't clear then, it's clear now how many people loved Blake.

A Facebook page has been created and filled with memories, along with thousands who are lending their support to Blake's family and friends. A video on that page shows Blake's locker at school, filled with messages from fellow students. Heather is also taking comfort in letters, written by friends and strangers.

"*You were such a caring, sweet and silly person who could put a smile on anyone's face,*" one letter's author said. Given that support, Boothe is now standing up. She wants others to see Blake's story and speak up, pay attention, and keep another kid from feeling like it's too much. She hopes to spread that message in Blake's memory.

"I'm fighting for kids out there that are like my son. This shouldn't have happened," Boothe said.

Blake was a student at Westfield Middle School. Fox 59 reached out to the district and was told it has provided crisis counseling to his classmates and passed information on to Westfield Police regarding his death.

A Westfield Police spokesman told Fox 59 the department conducted a standard death investigation and found no crime connected to his death.

http://fox59.com/2014/03/21/mothers-speaks-out-after-teens-suicide-hopes-his-memory-spurs-change/#axzz2x8PDLP00

About Teen Suicide

There are several complex reasons behind a suicide attempt by a teen. A rapid increase has been observed in suicide rates and attempts among adolescents. The suicide risk increases even more when adolescents have direct access to firearms and guns at home. In United the States, 60% of suicides among teens are committed with guns. Another commonly followed method among teens for attempting suicide is by overdosing on prescribed, non-prescribed and OTC medications. Suicide rates vary among girls and boys. It is seen that girls think twice before committing suicide as compared to boys.

Are you at risk for attempting suicide?

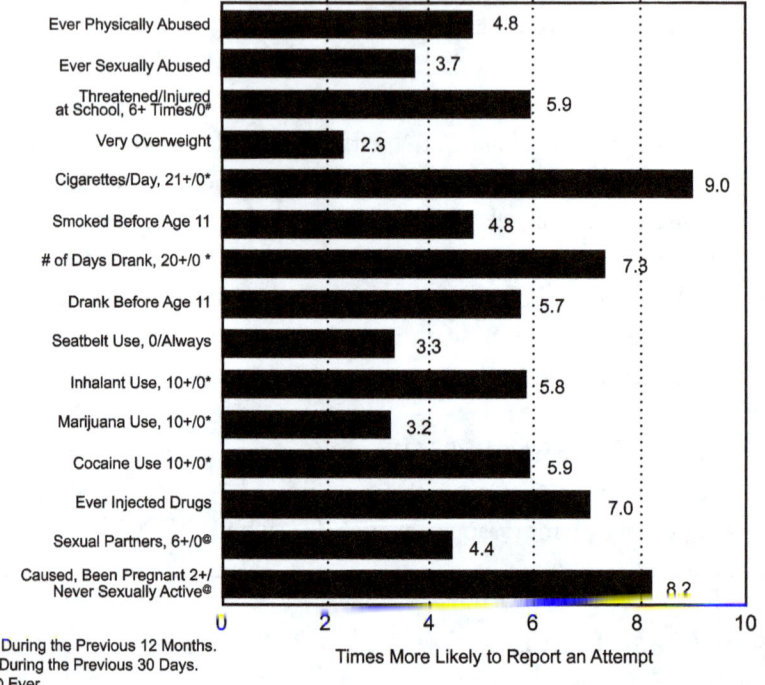

Figure 10. Odds of Reporting Having Made a Suicide Attempt During the Previous Year, by Selected Risk Factors, Oregon High School Students, 1997

\# During the Previous 12 Months.
* During the Previous 30 Days.
@ Ever.

- Teens suffering from mental problems, including depression, anxiety, insomnia, or bipolar disorders, are at greater risk of committing suicide.
- Teens facing major changes in life, such as parental separation, parents' divorce, any financial changes, etc., are also at high risk of contemplating committing suicide.
- Teens who are bullying victims are also at high risk of thinking about attempting suicide.
- Stress is one of the leading causes of low productivity, health issues, and psychological impairment. If not controlled appropriately, it can also lead to suicide in teens.

- A variety of research studies have already proved that low or impaired sleep affects mental and physical well-being. Inadequate sleep increases the secretion of stress hormones like cortisol and epinephrine, which leads to high cardiac activity and high glucose concentration. Teens who have sleeping problems (sleep disorders or insomnia) are 5 times more likely to attempt suicide.
- History of violence, domestic abuse, and sexual abuse at a younger age.
- History of psychological problems and depression in their family.
- Mood disorders or impulsive nature of teens also increases the risk of violence, depression, and self-harm.

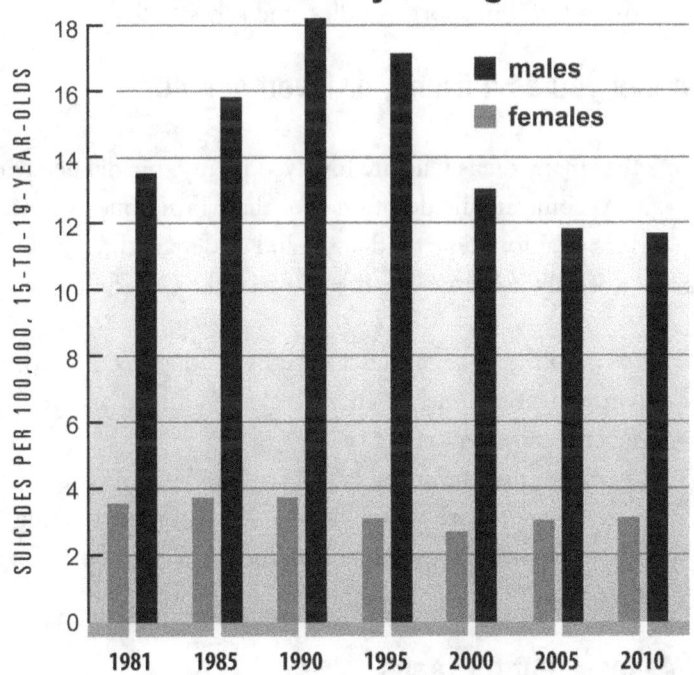

Warning Signs

Among teens, suicide often occurs due to any stressful event happening in life, like any school problems, death of a loved one, a divorce, break-up with significant other, or any major family conflict. Adolescents that start thinking about suicide may:

- Generally talks about death and suicide
- Talks all the time about feeling guilty or hopeless
- Give hints that they are going somewhere
- Keep themselves from family and friends' gatherings
- Write letters, poems, and songs of death
- Lose interest in their favorite activities or things
- Experience change in their sleeping habits
- Engage themselves in risky behaviors
- Lose interest in sports, studies, and school

What can you as a friend, or loved one do?

It seems that many teens who are involved in any suicidal behavior or who want to commit suicide often give their loved ones warning in advance. It is vital for teens to identify and understand those warning signs and possibly help save the life of a friend or loved one.

- It is important to watch for signs of depression. Keep the communication lines open with them, and express your love, concern, and support.
- If he/she is not comfortable talking with you, then suggest any neutral person with whom he/she is comfortable talking to.
- Try to help solve the problem, and seek the support and advice of an adult.

Self-Assessment for teens:

1. What are the factors that lead to teen suicide?

2. How can you help and/or support teen friends who are at risk of committing suicide?
3. What are the risk factors that increase the likelihood of suicide in teens?
4. How can you manage bullying?

Community Service, Meditation, and Success Principles

You may find vision and goals totally irrelevant and unnecessary to discuss with meditation and community service, but there is a reason why these subjects are discussed as a unit here.

***Amanda**, daughter of a Christian family, was active in church-related activities ever since she was a child. Growing up as a teen and being a high school student didn't really changed her practice.*

Her life was pretty organized and she always felt happiness while helping others. In fact, seeing other people satisfied was one of her goals and sources of motivation.

*On the other hand, her classmate **Tisha** is a troubled teen. Both of her parents work full time, leaving no one to take care of her. She spends most of her time watching movies, going out with friends, and lately she has started using drugs too.*

Where do you expect to see both girls in ten years?

Most importantly, what can possibly go wrong with both of them?

Amanda's life is pretty satisfying and rewarding; her parents, friends, and community like her. On the other hand, Tisha is more likely to:

- Perform poorly at school
- Drop out of high school
- Get involved in gang fights
- More likely to die from a drug overdose

- More likely to get permanently disabled due to driving under intoxication
- More likely to be disliked by her community and parents.

The rejection can lead to depression, violence, and even self-harm.

Self- Assessment in Teens

1. How can you volunteer for productive teen activities?
2. What are some of the volunteer activities in which you are interested?
3. How can volunteering protect and prevent you from teen social issues?

COMMUNITY SERVICE

Volunteer activities are exceptionally helpful in managing and improving social responsibilities in teens. When you involve yourself in constructive and positive habits, you make better use of your time and efforts.

Here are other benefits that you can gain from volunteer activities.

- Manage depression, anxiety, and other psychological disorders by seeing and interacting with people who are living in even worse living conditions. Helping others in need helps evoke and strengthen one's sense of self-worth and self-respect
- Improves your problem solving, multi-tasking, and social skills
- A higher likelihood to gain more respect and love from the community that may help in boosting confidence
- Getting experience and learning different skill-sets before actually starting a real job
- Volunteering also helps you to put your knowledge, skill-set, and academic learning into practice
- Provides you the ability and opportunities to network and communicate with other people

- Helps in improving the community and environment around you
- Promotes decision making and management skills
- Keeps you entertained, physically active, motivated, energized, and satisfied.

MEDITATION

There are several benefits of meditation. Being a teenager is often stressful (especially considering all the potential stressors like academic performance, physical activities, managing relationships, peer pressure, community expectations, and other issues).

Likewise, it is also clear that in the absence of any constructive stress relieving options, such as meditation, the chances of living a healthy and normal life decreases substantially.

Among the several benefits of meditation, some notable ones are:

- Development of mental and spiritual strength
- Development of mental and interpersonal skills, such as intuition, wisdom, and creativity
- Ability to identify, sort out, and solve issues
- Improves physical strength and forces
- Enhance physical, sexual, and emotional relationships
- Helps in optimal development of reality and nature

There are numerous other benefits that are listed below in the table:

Benefits of Meditation

If all that is not enough for you, we know the benefits of taking time to meditate include:

- Lower Heart Rate
- Lower Levels of Stress and Cortisol (and we know stress leads to illness)

- More Focus on What is Important
- More Effective communication with Others
- Sleep Better
- Support Weight Loss
- Process Pain and Emotions More Effectively
- Lowers Risk of Depression
- Lowers Blood Pressure
- Decrease rate of Aging

How do you meditate?

There are several techniques, postures, and tips that can be employed. I suggest you start with a simple posture and develop a habit or routine first (by allocating some time from your daily routine, regardless of your activities or time availability).

If you are satisfied with the results, you can always go ahead and do other postures and adopt other techniques as well.

Here are a few basic postures

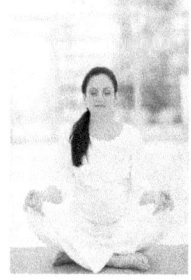 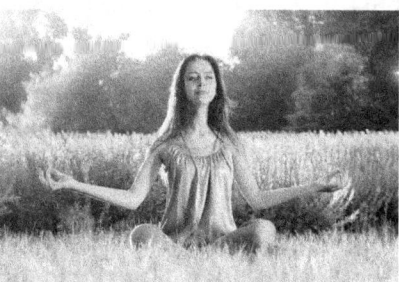 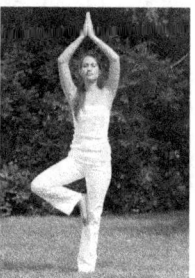

Start with any one and allocate at least 15 to 25 minutes each day for meditation.

For best results:

- Set one place/ spot for meditation
- Choose preferably morning or late evening for meditation (or any time you feel you can concentrate)
- Include friends and family members as well in your meditation plan
- Be creative, innovative, and consistent

PRINCIPLES FOR SUCCESS

18-year-old John is always over-occupied with being better and improving himself. He is a nice charming young man and unlike most teens his age, he is exploring ways that can make him successful and rich.

Wait a minute—is being successful and being rich synonymous (the same thing)?

Obviously not!

A person who knows how to control himself, his anger, agitation, frustration, and anxiety is successful; however, monetary compensation does not always follow success.

Knowing principles for success can make you a stronger, likable person, and eventually money flows too. However, setting a target of being rich can neither make you strong nor rich or wealthy.

Teen Success Principles:

12 Principles for Success

1. *Be yourself, no matter what*
2. *Set high standards, and don't settle*
3. *Change any limiting beliefs*
4. *Model strategies that work, because success leaves clues*

5. *Do not compete with others, because there is not competition*
6. *Identify your weaknesses and work on improving them*
7. *Learn new skills and refine old ones*
8. *Follow the right path, no matter how hard it is*
9. *Don't be afraid of making mistakes; everyone makes them*
10. *Take accountability and responsibility for your actions*
11. *Love and respect others*
12. *Give way more than you take*

What can stop you from achieving success?

1. Angst (a feeling of anxiety):

Sandra is a very sensitive 16-year-old female. Ever since childhood, she was always worried about other people around her. But isn't it a good thing that she has a caring heart?

   Well, Sandra was an extreme case before seeking help. She used to obsess a lot on circumstances, situations, and other negative happenings around her (or perhaps anywhere in the world).

> Well, your symptoms are consistant with a heavy case of Angst. Luckily this is the treatable kind, a sub-malaise known as Teenage Angst. Treatment includes ten years of experience and a loss of purity and ideals.

At times, when we feel negatively about bullies, mean kids, or other fearful events, however, oftentimes being extra sensitive can also compromise your development and success. Learn to love yourself and always remember that only YOU can help your own self.

People like Sandra should learn to channel their negativity about the world in a positive direction. Direct their fear to the path of confidence and instead of feeling bad about people (and harming your health), it is better to be a part of volunteer programs and actually help those in need.

2. Anxiety:

Anxiety is a normal emotion as long as it is controlled.

You can get anxious before getting the result of your finals or when you meet someone. However, your anxiety is getting out of hand if:

- You are experiencing trouble sleeping
- Maintaining day-to-day relationships
- If you are developing physical signs or complications of anxiety, like headaches, muscle aches, fear, depression, body aches, etc.

Success is impossible unless you learn to control and rule your emotions and weaknesses.

Complications of uncontrolled anxiety and depression in Teens:

As a teen, you should understand that unnecessary worrying can compromise your goals and success. Here are a proven set of complications of poorly managed anxiety in teens:

- Impaired judgment that increases the risk of making bad decisions

- Loss of appetite and poor mental and physical health
- High risk of developing dependency on drugs / alcohol
- Indecisiveness
- Apprehension
- Loss of confidence

Anger:

Anger, aggression and agitation are normal feelings or emotions. We all get angry at different points in time. However, being angry means controlling yourself and solving the cause of your anger.

How do most teens take out their anger?

Some cry and others punch walls, while others just remain calm and quiet. Well, all three behaviors are extreme—a better strategy is to approach the situation wisely and prevent it from happening.

You can also exercise, meditate, or perform yoga to channel your anger in a positive direction.

Here is a real story of what anger can do to you. This news story is about Sean Hackett.

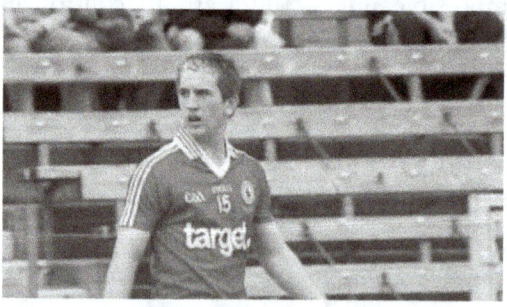

The former captain of the Tyrone minor football team murdered his father Aloysius (Wishie) Hackett on January 4, 2013 at their family home in Co Tyrone.

His mother Eilis wept as she sat behind him in the packed public gallery of Dungannon Crown Court. The 19-year-old had always admitted the unlawful killing of his father, whom he shot twice in the head in the driveway of their Aghindarrah Road family home in Augher.

It took the jury of six women and six men just over two-and-a-half hours to reach a verdict.

Initially, there was some confusion over the not guilty murder verdict and trial judge Mr. Justice Stephens asked the jury to retire.

Within moments, he called them back to ask if "all of you" had reached a verdict in relation to the alternative charge of manslaughter and diminished responsibility. The foreperson said they had reached a guilty verdict on the charge.

Afterwards, Mr. Justice Stephens remanded the teenager back into custody until further reports on him are obtained and he is sentenced next month. The jury accepted the defense's case that Hackett was a mentally disturbed teenager on the possible verge of schizophrenia when he killed his father.

During the trial, the jury was told that Hackett, who was armed with a Czech hunting rifle, waited for his father. He had borrowed the rifle from a friend. A former chairman of St. Macartan's GAA club, Hackett's father was returning home from a meeting that evening.

When he saw his son holding the gun, he yelled "no!" But as he fell to the ground, his son had already re-loaded the rifle, and fired again. Hackett, after killing his father, went to him and said a prayer while holding his hand.

The court heard that when first questioned, he told police "something was wrong at the house," possibly a burglary, but later admitted: "I did it... I shot him."

Later in a prepared statement, he reported: *"I was involved in an incident with reference to the death of my daddy whom I love very much... I have been suffering from depression and was seeking medical attention at the time. That's all I have to say at this time."*

His mother, in utter sadness, told the press that her son is a great guy and although she has always been very proud of him, she has no idea why he did what he did.

Psychiatrist Dr. Fred Browne said Hackett was suffering from *"an adjustment disorder" brought on by the break-up with his girlfriend, but that could in no way excuse or explain his homicidal tendencies and the feeling of power, excitement, and control he got from the thoughts of killing a parent.*

Source: http://www.rte.ie/news/2014/0306/600487-aloysius-hackett/

Arrogance:

Arrogance is a negative behavior that eats away the positive in you. Arrogance tells you that you are superior and invincible. In fact, very interestingly, when teens think they are being confident, they are usually being arrogant.

But why is arrogance so bad?

Arrogance is a form of ignorance. It affects your capacity and capability to learn new things, admit mistakes, and work towards improvement.

If you don't improve yourself or learn from your mistakes, you are much more likely to repeat the mistakes and perhaps harm yourself quite badly someday.

Here is a summary of the success principles that in my opinion can help you in becoming a better person.

Say NO to…	Say YES to….
Jealousy	Kindness and generosity
Arrogance and attitude	Self-respect and confidence
Profanity and violence	Secret keeping and trustworthy
Self-indulgence, self-centeredness and selfishness	Friendship and respect
Stealing	Love, care, and self-control
Cheating and lying	Humility and honor
	Truth and responsibility

Helping others and realizing the needs and requirements of other people is an essential part of learning and being successful. A simple act, such as donating your unwanted clothing, shoes, games, etc., can benefit others who may be less fortunate or experiencing hard times.

Here is what Nicholas Lowinger did.

Teenager Nicholas Lowinger Gives Thousands of Shoes to Homeless

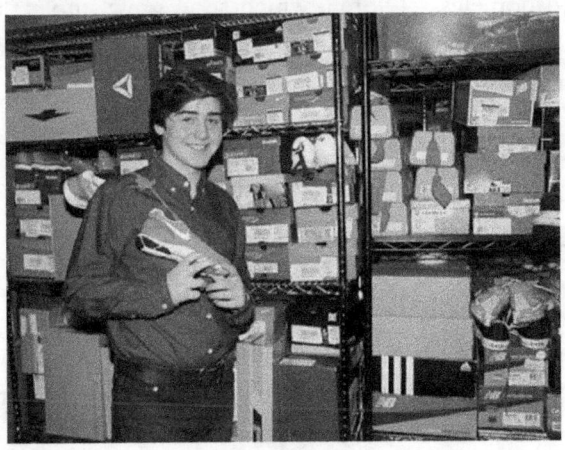

Brittany Taylor, 28, was fired from her job at a grocery store where she was working for the last 15 years. The incident took place just before Thanksgiving Eve. Due to a lack of any potential savings that could save her from a sudden blow in rainy days, she soon found herself at a homeless shelter in frosty Providence, R.I. with two children John, 7, and Johneya, 5.

Children's shoes were among the many needs that the shelter couldn't fulfill. With the approach of a snowy winter, Johneya only had flat, ballet-style shoes that were already peeling, and John's sneakers were already destroyed.

Yet, before the harsh winter could harm the little flowers, the children did get new sneakers and winter boots courtesy of local teen Nicholas Lowinger. The owner of Gotta Have Sole foundation has distributed more than 16,000 pairs of footwear in more than 32 states.

Sixteen-year-old Nicholas said his interest in helping needy homeless children developed at the age of 5, when his parents took him to a homeless shelter. He realized that the happiness of getting a new pair of footwear with lights turned to sympathy for those who had nothing to wear.

Nicholas started donating his old footwear to homeless shelters, but appreciated the fact that oftentimes it is not very comfortable to wear shoes broken in by someone else. So he created a community service project to donate new shoes to homeless children, which soon grew into a national operation with several shoe retailers (including 6pm, Walmart, Timberland, and Stride Rite) as sponsors.

A Homespun Operation

The headquarters of the operation is the Lowinger family garage in Cranston, R.I. The venture's functioning is very well-organized. Shelters provide orders for shoes, and the young growing foundation and its volunteers fill these orders by using shoes provided by sponsors. If he doesn't have the right shoes handy, Nicholas will buy them, using cash donations. If the shelters are local, Nicholas will hand out the shoes in person.

The gift packages include socks and personalized messages by Nicholas on cards shaped like shoes: "This is a gift because you're worthy."

Nicholas is also trying to change people's perceptions and sentiments regarding homeless people who have fallen on hard times.

Gotta Have Sole has chapters in Florida, Connecticut, Massachusetts, and South Carolina, with a rotating roster of roughly 2,000 volunteers participating at any given time.

Rachael Kaplan, 38, who brought her children to Nicholas's home to volunteer is one of several moms in Rhode Island. Madelyn, her daughter, was 6 the first time she volunteered (she's now 9 and continues to volunteer), and Kaplan wanted to "teach her to feel lucky with what she has." They picked up one of the many orders sent to Gotta Have Sole, had Madelyn buy shoes that her family paid for, and brought the shoes to Nicholas, who explained what he was trying to do. Madelyn also helped design and write several cards.

"Through opportunities like that, we are becoming better people," Kaplan says.

In February 2014 after children were killed in the Newtown shootings, Nicholas received a Charlotte Bacon Act of Kindness Award.

Nicholas told the crowd after accepting the award: "I just have a challenge to all of you … to find some way to be a kinder person or be a peacemaker, and make the world a better place. I think there's a peacemaker in all of us."

http://www.people.com/people/article/0,,20800344,00.html

Activity

- *Make a list of your potential stressors and relaxers?*
- *How can you manage your stress?*
- *How do you actually manage your stress?*
- *What are 2-3 success principles you can start applying today?*
- *What are some ways you can help others (by giving of your time, unwanted items or resources)?*
- *How do you rate yourself on a scale of 1-10 in the management of anger, anxiety, and stress?*

CHAPTER 10
RIGHTS AS A TEEN WHEN SEEKING HEALTHCARE

Don't you hate it when everyone treats you like a kid (although you believe that you are a grown up)?

Growing up means additional responsibility and accountability, yet how can you act responsible when you are not allowed to make decisions regarding your own well-being?

If this is what you think, here is what you should know…

As a teenager, you can make decisions about your health and well-being (as an independent individual) without requiring any consent from your parents. Here is a recent example…

A pregnant teen will be able to give birth to her baby against her parent's wishes

According to court documents, a 16-year-old girl represented by attorneys was granted a long-term injunction against her parents in a Texas family court.

The injunction will last for the duration of her pregnancy. She is currently 10 weeks pregnant.

The girl has been given permission by the court to use her car to go to school, work, and medical appointments as part of the order. As stated in the court documents, the parents of the teen took away the car as part of their effort to force the teen to get an abortion.

In addition, the parents of teen are also liable to pay for half of the hospital bill after she gives birth; however, they don't have any obligation if the teen is married to the baby's 16-year-old biological father.

Greg Terra, president of the Texas Center for Defense of Life, said in a blog post on the group's website:

"We are extremely happy with the judge's decision today and we are very proud of our teenage client for being strong enough to stand against her parents to save her unborn child's life."

Attorneys filed the case on the behalf of the teen this month. She argued that her parents "are violating her federal constitutional rights to carry her child to term by coercing her to have an abortion with both verbal and physical threats and harassment."

The attorney explained that various such cases have been presented in the court of law and verdicts have always supported the teen.

"These girls are in a bind, particularly in a situation where their parents are forcing them to do something they don't want to do," Casey said. "Regardless of the [situation], that's her parents and she should expect support from them in this situation, not resentment and anger."

When the pregnancy was confirmed, the teenager's father allegedly *"became extremely angry, was insistent that R.E.K. was not having the baby, and that the decision was not up to her,* according to the lawsuit. He stated he was going to take her to have an abortion and that the decision was his, end of story."

The teen explained in the lawsuit that the parents took her phone and forced her to abandon school and take two jobs (with no car) in an effort to *"make her miserable so that she would give in to the coercion and have the abortion."*

Inspired from: http://abcnews.go.com/blogs/headlines/2013/02/texas-teen-wins-right-to-give-birth-over-parents-objections/

Teenagers (above the age of 13) are classified as minors, which suggests in many cases that they have less responsibility and are bound to their parental or guardian assistance. Yet you can seek medical or healthcare services as an adult without having to worry about parental consent.

In fact, your information will be kept confidential in the same manner as that of adults.

What should you know about your rights to healthcare services as a teen?

As a teen, you have the right to seek confidential and completely private treatment and advice without your parents' knowledge about these issues:

- Seeking treatment for HIV, hepatitis, or other sexually transmitted diseases
- Seeking knowledge about contraceptive options
- Getting condoms or contraceptive devices
- Prenatal check-ups and maintaining teen pregnancy
- Right to make the decision individually to keep or abort the baby
- In seeking advice, sharing information and getting help from a healthcare provider about potential sexual or physical abuse from a partner or stranger (in some parts of the world, healthcare providers are required to notify the state and parents if the child is underage or if the risk of future abuse is present)
- If you have question or concerns about sexuality or sexual orientation
- If you want to know more about drugs, risk of addiction, help for addiction, or other similar issues
- If you seek help or assistance regarding screening for sexually transmitted diseases

What are the limitations of confidential teen healthcare services?

Although optimal relief and confidentiality protect teens by law, if expensive treatment is required, he/she will ultimately have to seek parental consent and support (both for financial and non-financial reasons). In either case, healthcare providers don't notify parents unless you supervise and/or permit them to.

If you require a major surgery (or chemotherapy), decisions in most parts of the world are made by parents (or healthcare professionals that represent the interest of the patient and state).

Some other instances when your healthcare provider has the right to breach the patient confidentiality agreement are:

- If your healthcare provider strongly feels that you are incompetent or unable to understand the complete details of the procedure or illness
- If you are potentially making a decision that may endanger your life
- If you are younger than 16 and are maintaining sexual relations with someone who is over 21
- If you are 14 or younger and are engaged in sexual relations with anyone above the age of 14

Why is it important for you to know about your medical rights?

- As a teenager, does it make any difference to you if your parents are notified each time you seek medical help for screening or management of sexually transmitted diseases?
- How likely are you to seek psychiatric care if you are not sure that your healthcare professional will keep this information confidential?

- Would you seek the advice, assistance, or guidance of a healthcare professional for birth control pills or contraception if you require parental consent for this information?

When the same questions were asked in multiple surveys, the results were pretty disappointing. More than 50% of teens responded negatively to these questions, which is understandable since most teens feel reluctant to share discrete information about their sex life with their parents.

Here is a list of all the healthcare services you may seek without having parental consent.

WOMEN'S SEXUAL AND REPRODUCTIVE HEALTH	ADDITIONAL WOMEN'S HEALTH CARE	MEN'S SEXUAL HEALTH
• Contraceptive counseling, services and methods (as prescribed for women) • Numerous potential health services • HIV AND STI counseling • STI testing (HIV, chlamydia, gonorrhea, syphilis) • Cervical cancer screening (Pap testing and HPV testing) • HPV vaccination • Hepatitis A and B vaccination	• Well-women visits • Domestic and interpersonal violence screening and counseling • Breast cancer prevention mammography, genetic screening and counseling, and chemoprevention counseling	• HIV AND STI counseling • STI testing (HIV, chlamydia, gonorrhea, syphilis) • Hepatitis A and B vaccination

Since the laws in different parts of the world may vary, you should ideally check with your healthcare professional before making a final decision regarding seeking medical help.

Self-Assessment for teens

- What do you understand about teens' rights to healthcare services?
- How much do you know about the healthcare rules, regulations, and laws in your state or region?

CONCLUSION

To sum up:

Being an adolescent is the most exciting phase of a person's life. With so many hormonal, physiological, psychological, and biochemical changes happening in the body, as well as all the new responsibilities that are added to your daily routine and exposure to so many new substances (both good and bad), it is logical to understand that being a teenager or adolescent is a roller-coaster ride.

You are subjected to peer pressure, face dating related issues and possibly experience violence, discrimination, or neglect. Young adolescents are more likely to be influenced by the wrong crowd, illicit substances, and other negative temptations, but having a resourceful guide such as literature, parental guidance, and teachers' assistance can definitely prove helpful in reducing the chances of succumbing to common difficulties and problems.

This book is designed to bring to your attention some of the very common issues that are faced by adolescents and productive solutions to manage the issues positively. Once again, it is very important to seek help and assistance whenever you feel that something is not right.

Feel free to take notes, share with friends and learn to assess and differentiate the right from the wrong if you want to emerge as a strong, responsible, and successful adult.

Remember, you control your destiny, so "Take Charge" of your health and life TODAY!

I wish you all the best in your youthfulness and years ahead.

RESOURCES

Academy for Eating Disorders

- Provides leadership in eating disorders research, education, treatment, and prevention.
- Disseminates knowledge regarding eating disorders to members of the academy, other professionals, and the general public.
http://www.aedweb.org

Academy of Nutrition and Dietetics

- Works to serve the public through the promotion of optimal nutrition, health, and well-being.
http://www.eatright.org

American Academy of Pediatrics

- Provides information and publications to promote the health, safety, and well-being of infants, children, adolescents, and young adults.
http://www.aap.org

American College of Sports Medicine

- Provides publications, audiotapes, and videotapes on physical fitness and weight loss to health professionals and the general public.
http://www.acsm.org

American Diabetes Association (ADA)

- Provides information to the public on diabetes and related topics, including nutrition, exercise, and treatment.
- ADA also offers patient referrals.
- Operators and information are available in Spanish. http://www.diabetes.org

American Heart Association

- Features a free online walking guide, physical activity and nutrition tracker, healthy recipes, and sample stretches. http://www.mystartonline.org

American Public Health Association

- Serves the public through its scientific and practice programs, publications, educational services, and advocacy efforts. http://www.apha.org

BAM! Body and Mind

- This interactive website provides information to help you move more and eat better. It includes games, daily tips, and trivia questions. http://www.bam.gov

Best Bones Forever!

- This bone health campaign encourages girls and their friends to grow stronger together and stay strong forever. http://www.bestbonesforever.gov

Calorie Control Council

- This site allows users to calculate the number of calories burned during physical activity.
  http://www.caloriecontrol.org/exercalc.html

Center for Nutrition Policy and Promotion

- Provides information about nutrition and food selection, *including* dietary guidelines and healthy eating plans.
  http://www.cnpp.usda.gov

Center for Science in the Public Interest

- This interactive questionnaire helps users determine whether they make healthy food choices at restaurants.
  http://www.cspinet.org/nah/quiz/index.html

Dietary Guidelines for Americans, 2010

- The healthy eating content in *Take Charge* is based on these guidelines.
  http://www.health.gov/dietaryguidelines

Food and Drug Administration (FDA)

- Provides information and publications about food products and dietary supplements to health professionals and the public.
  http://www.fda.gov

Center for Food Safety and Applied Nutrition

- Provides information and publications about food products and dietary supplements to health professionals and the public.
  http://www.fda.gov/Food/default.htm

Center for Drug Evaluation and Research (CDER)

Human Drug Information
- Provides information and publications on drug-related subjects to health professionals and the public.
http://www.fda.gov/Drugs/default.htm

Girlshealth.gov

- This federal resource provides girls with reliable health information on physical activity, nutrition, stress reduction, and more.
http://www.girlshealth.gov

Health Power for Minorities

- Through its website, helps minority populations identify resources for health information.
http://www.healthpowerforminorities.com

International Food Information Council

- This site promotes healthy eating and physical activity among children and their parents.
http://kidnetic.com

Let's Move!

- This campaign inspires children and teens to get moving. Visit the website to read tips and take action.
http://www.letsmove.gov

Media-Smart Youth

- Media-Smart Youth: Eat, Think, and Be Active! is an interactive after-school program that informs young people about the media's influence on food and physical activity choices.
  http://www.nichd.nih.gov/msy

MyPlate

- MyPlate offers more information, tips, and interactive tools to help you make a plan for moving more and eating better.
  http://www.ChooseMyPlate.gov

National Center for Complementary and Alternative

- *Medicine (NCCAM)* Conducts and supports research and training. Disseminates information on complementary and alternative medicine to practitioners and the public.
  http://nccam.nih.gov

National Diabetes Education Program (NDEP)

NDEP
- provides teens with information about diabetes. The website offers publications and resources on how teens can prevent and manage diabetes.
  http://www.yourdiabetesinfo.org

National Institute of Mental Health

- Provides information about mental health, including eating disorders, to health professionals and the public.
- Develops, identifies, and distributes educational materials.
  http://www.nimh.nih.gov

National Health Information Center

- A health information referral service that puts health professionals and consumers who have health questions in touch with those organizations that are best able to provide answers.
  http://www.health.gov/NHIC

National Heart, Lung, and Blood Institute

- This site allows users to calculate their body mass index, or BMI.
  http://www.nhlbi.nih.gov/guidelines/obesity/BMI/bmicalc.htm

National Organization for Rare Disorders

- Provides information on rare disorders to health professionals and the public. Maintains the Rare Disease Database.
  http://www.rarediseases.org

Nutrition.gov

- This website provides reader-friendly information on a number of topics related to healthy eating.
  http://www.nutrition.gov

Obesity Action Coalition (OAC)

- Offers free educational resources on obesity, morbid obesity, and childhood obesity, in addition to consequences of and treatments for these conditions.
- Conducts a variety of advocacy efforts throughout the United States on both the national and state levels and encourages individuals to become proactive advocates.
  http://www.obesityaction.org

Office of Minority Health

- Provides the general public, health professionals, the media, and Congress with up-to-date, science-based information on weight control, obesity, physical activity, and related nutritional issues.
  http://minorityhealth.hhs.gov

Portion Distortion Quiz

- This quiz on the website of the National Heart, Lung, and Blood Institute shows how portion sizes have changed over time.
  http://hp2010.nhlbihin.net/portion

President's Challenge

- The President's Challenge encourages you to make physical activity a regular part of life.
  http://www.fitness.gov/participate-in-programs/presidents-challenge

School Nutrition Association (SNA)

- Helps its more than 55,000 school nutrition professional members provide high-quality, low-cost meals to students across the country.
- Offers materials that promote school nutrition programs and healthy school meals.
  http://www.schoolnutrition.org

Strategies to Overcome and Prevent (STOP) Obesity Alliance

- Works to reverse the nation's obesity trend and related conditions such as diabetes and heart disease.
- Researches barriers to weight loss and healthy weight.

- Offers guides to help parents discuss weight and health with their children, as well as obesity fact sheets.
  http://www.stopobesityalliance.org

Take Off Pounds Sensibly (TOPS) Club

- Provides weight-loss support and education on healthy eating and regular physical activity.
- Sponsors research to find obesity's root cause and treatment.
- Offers materials and weekly support meetings in many states.
  http://www.tops.org

The Obesity Society

- Promotes education, research, and community action to improve the quality of life for people with obesity.
- Develops, extends, and disseminates knowledge in the field of obesity.
  http://www.obesity.org

Team Nutrition

- Team Nutrition focuses on the role nutritious school meals, nutrition education, and a health-promoting school environment play in helping you learn to enjoy healthy eating and physical activity.
  http://www.fns.usda.gov/tn/about.html

United States Department of Agriculture

- Provides leadership on food, agriculture, natural resources, and related issues based on sound public policy, the best available science, and efficient management.
- The USDA Center for Nutrition Policy and Promotion releases the Dietary Guidelines for Americans every 5 years.

The *2010 Dietary Guidelines for Americans* can be found online at http://health.gov/dietaryguidelines.
- Consumers are encouraged to refer to the newly released *2008 Physical Activity Guidelines for Americans*, released by the U.S. Department of Health and Human Services. The Guidelines can be found online at http://www.health.gov/paguidelines.

USDA's Team Nutrition

USDA Food and Nutrition Service
- Focuses on the role nutritious school meals, nutrition education, and a health-promoting school environment play in helping students learn to enjoy healthy eating and physical activity. http://teamnutrition.usda.gov

U.S. Department of Agriculture

- This site provides a directory of current listing of farmers markets throughout the United States. http://search.ams.usda.gov/farmersmarkets

U.S. Department of Agriculture Center for Nutrition Policy and Promotion

- Visitors to this site receive personalized eating plans based on height, weight, sex, and age. There are specific sections for adults and children. http://www.choosemyplate.gov

We Can!

We Can! Provides information to caregivers and community members so they may help children and teens stay healthy. *http://www.nhlbi.nih.gov/health/public/heart/obesity/wecan/index.htm*

Weight Control Information Network (WIN)

- An information service of the National Institute of Diabetes and Digestive and Kidney Disease (NIDDK) http://win.niddk.nih.gov/publications/take_charge.htm

2008 Physical Activity Guidelines for Americans

- These guidelines general information on physical activity for teenagers, including how often you should be active and which activities are best for you.
  http://www.health.gov/PAGuidelines

BMI calculation made easy:

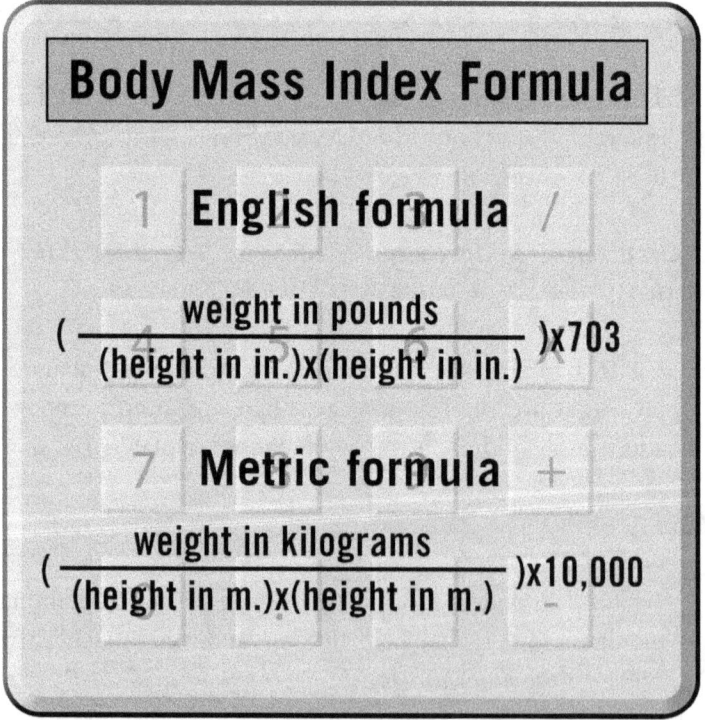

BMI Table

You can also determine your BMI using the table below. First, identify your weight (to the nearest 10 pounds) in one of the columns across the top, then move your finger down the column until you come to the row that represents your height. Inside the square where your weight and height meet is a number that is an estimate of your BMI. For example, if you weigh 160 pounds and are 5'7", your BMI is 25. The numbers in bold mean you are classified as being obese.

HEIGHT	WEIGHT														
	100	110	120	130	140	150	160	170	180	190	200	210	220	230	240	250
5'0"	20	21	23	25	21	29	**31**	**33**	**35**	**37**	**39**	**41**	**43**	**45**	**47**	**49**
5'1"	19	21	23	25	26	28	**30**	**32**	**34**	**36**	**38**	**40**	**42**	**43**	**45**	**47**
5'2"	18	20	22	24	26	27	29	**31**	**33**	**35**	**37**	**38**	**40**	**42**	**44**	**46**
5'3"	18	19	21	23	25	27	28	**30**	**32**	**34**	**35**	**37**	**39**	**41**	**43**	**44**
5'4"	17	19	21	22	24	26	27	29	**31**	**33**	**34**	**36**	**38**	**39**	**41**	**43**
5'5"	17	18	20	22	23	25	27	28	**30**	**32**	**33**	**35**	**37**	**38**	**40**	**42**
5'6"	16	18	19	21	23	24	26	27	29	**31**	**32**	**34**	**36**	**37**	**39**	**40**
5'7"	16	17	19	20	22	23	25	27	28	**30**	**31**	**33**	**34**	**36**	**38**	**39**
5'8"	15	17	18	20	21	23	24	26	27	29	**30**	**32**	**33**	**35**	**36**	**38**
5'9"	15	16	18	19	21	22	24	25	27	28	**30**	**31**	**32**	**34**	**35**	**37**
5'10"	14	16	17	19	20	22	23	24	26	27	29	**30**	**32**	**33**	**34**	**36**
5'11"	14	15	17	18	20	21	22	24	25	26	27	28	**30**	**32**	**33**	**35**
6'0"	14	15	16	18	19	20	22	23	24	26	27	28	**30**	**31**	**33**	**34**
6'1"	13	15	16	17	18	20	21	22	24	25	26	28	29	**30**	**32**	**33**
6'2"	13	14	15	17	18	19	21	22	23	24	26	27	28	**30**	**31**	**32**
6'3"	12	14	15	16	17	19	20	21	22	24	25	26	27	29	**30**	**31**
6'4"	12	13	15	16	17	18	19	21	22	23	24	26	27	28	29	**30**

http://www.health.harvard.edu/topic/BMI-Calculator

Glycemic Index and Glycemic Load of Popular Foods

Bold = Low Glycemic Index and Glycemic Load

Type of Food	Glycemic Index	Serving Size	Net Carbs	Glycemic Load
Peanuts	**14**	4 oz (113g)	15	**2**
Bean sprouts	**25**	1 cup (104g)	4	**1**
Grapefruits	**25**	½ large (166g)	11	**3**
Pizza	**30**	2 slices (260g)	42	13
Lowfat yogurt	**33**	1 cup (245g)	47	16
Apples	**38**	1 medium (138g)	16	**6**
Spaghetti	**42**	1 cup (140g)	38	16
Carrots	47	1 large (72g)	5	**2**
Oranges	48	1 medium (131g)	12	**6**
Bananas	52	1 large (136g)	27	16
Potato chips	54	4 oz (114g)	55	30
Snickers Bar	55	1 bar (113g)	64	35
Brown rice	55	1 cup (195g)	42	23
Honey	55	1 tbsp (21g)	17	**9**
Oatmeal	58	1 cup (234g)	21	12
Ice cream	61	1 cup (72g)	16	10
Macaroni and cheese	54	1 serving (166g)	47	30
Raisins	64	1 small box (43g)	32	20
White rice	64	1 cup (186g)	52	33
Sugar (sucrose)	68	1 tbsp (12g)	12	**8**
White bread	70	1 slice (30g)	14	10
Watermelon	72	1 cup (154g)	11	**8**
Popcorn	72	2 cups (16g)	10	**7**
Baked potato	85	1 medium (173g)	33	28
Glucose	100	(50g)	50	50

REFERENCES

1. http://www.nami.org/Template.cfm?Section=By_Illness&template=/ContentManagement/ContentDisplay.cfm&ContentID=88551
2. http://jasonfoundation.com/prp/facts/youth-suicide-statistics/
3. http://www.cdc.gov/chronicdisease/overview/index.htm
4. Wu, S.Y., & Green, A. (2000). *Projection of chronic illness prevalence and cost inflation.* Santa Monica, CA: RAND Health.
5. Ogden, C.L., Carroll, M.D., & Flegal, K.M. (2008). High body mass index for age among US children and adolescents, 2003–2006. *Journal of the American Medical Association, 299,* 2401–2405.
6. http://www.advocatesforyouth.org/datingviolence
7. http://www.actforyouth.net/resources/rf/rf_romantic_0707.pdf
8. http://www.pamf.org/teen/abc/unhealthy/
9. http://www.breakthecycle.org/
10. http://www.healthyteennetwork.org/index.asp?Type=B_BASIC&SEC=%7B93D10D6F-011B-4718-AFF0-14836BE6098A%7D
11. http://www.anad.org/get-information/about-eating-disorders/eating-disorders-statistics/
12. Kohler, P. K., Manhart, L. E., & Lafferty, W. E. (2008). Abstinence-only and comprehensive sex education and the initiation of sexual activity and teen pregnancy. *Journal of Adolescent Health, 42*(4), 344-351.
13. Satin, A. J., Leveno, K. J., Sherman, M. L., Reedy, N. J., Lowe, T. W., & McIntire, D. D. (1994). Maternal youth and pregnancy outcomes: Middle school versus high school age

groups compared with women beyond the teen years. *American Journal of Obstetrics and Gynecology, 171*(1), 184-187.
14. Barber, N. (2000). On the relationship between country sex ratios and teen pregnancy rates: A replication. *Cross-Cultural Research, 34*(1), 26-37.
15. Santelli, J. S., Abma, J., Ventura, S., Lindberg, L., Morrow, B., Anderson, J. E., & Hamilton, B. E. (2004). Can changes in sexual behaviors among high school students explain the decline in teen pregnancy rates in the 1990s? *Journal of Adolescent Health, 35*(2), 80-90.
16. Finkelstein, D. M., Kubzansky, L. D., & Goodman, E. (2006). Social status, stress, and adolescent smoking. *Journal of Adolescent Health, 39*(5), 678-685.
17. Kobak, R. R., Sudler, N., & Gamble, W. (1991). Attachment and depressive symptoms during adolescence: A developmental pathways analysis. *Development and Psychopathology, 3*(4), 461-474.
18. Young, S. J., Ji, L. W., Chang, S. J., Fang, T. H., Hsueh, T. J., Meen, T. H., & Chen, I. C. (2007). Nanoscale mechanical characteristics of vertical ZnO nanowires grown on ZnO: Ga/glass templates. *Nanotechnology, 18*(22), 225603.
19. Black, M. M., & Nitz, K. (1996). Grandmother co-residence, parenting, and child development among low income, urban teen mothers. *Journal of Adolescent Health, 18*(3), 218-226.
20. Jaycox, Lisa H., Stein, B.D., Paddock, S., Miles, J.N.V., Chandra, A, Meredith, L.S., Tanielian, T., Hickey, S., & Burnam, M.A. (2009). Impact of teen depression on academic, social, and physical functioning. *Pediatrics,* 124(4), e596-e605.
21. McArt, E. W., Shulman, D.A., and Gajary, E. (1999). Developing an educational workshop on teen depression and suicide: a proactive community intervention. *Child Welfare,* 78(6).
22. Mellits, E. D., & Cheek, D. B. (1970). The assessment of body water and fatness from infancy to adulthood. *Monographs of the society for research in child development,* 12-26.

23. Esrey, S. A., & Habicht, J. P. (1986). Epidemiologic evidence for health benefits from improved water and sanitation in developing countries. *Epidemiologic Reviews, 8*, 117-128.
24. World Health Organization (Ed.). (2004). Guidelines for drinking-water quality: recommendations (Vol. 1). World Health Organization.
25. Berge, J. M., Wall, M., Larson, N., Loth, K. A., & Neumark-Sztainer, D. (2013). Family functioning: Associations with weight status, eating behaviors, and physical activity in adolescents. *Journal of Adolescent Health, 52*(3), 351-357.
26. Sirard, J. R., Bruening, M., Wall, M. M., Eisenberg, M. E., Kim, S. K., & Neumark-Sztainer, D. (2013). Physical activity and screen time in adolescents and their friends. *American Journal of Preventive Medicine, 44*(1), 48-55.
27. Horn, K., Branstetter, S., Zhang, J., Jarrett, T., O'Hara Tompkins, N., Anesetti-Rothermel, A., & Dino, G. (2013). Understanding physical activity outcomes as a function of teen smoking cessation. *Journal of Adolescent Health, 53*(1), 125-131.
28. Boyer, C. B., Shafer, M. A., Wibbelsman, C. J., Seeberg, D., Teitle, E., & Lovell, N. (2000). Associations of sociodemographic, psychosocial, and behavioral factors with sexual risk and sexually transmitted diseases in teen clinic patients. *Journal of Adolescent Health, 27*(2), 102-111.
29. Kirby, D., Lepore, G., & Ryan, J. (2005). Sexual risk and protective factors. Factors affecting teen sexual behavior pregnancy childbearing and sexually transmitted disease: Which are important? Which can you change?
30. Bunnell, R.E., Dahlberg, L., Rolfs, R., Ransom, R., Gershman, K., Farshy, C., Newhall, W.J., Schmid, S., Stone, K., and St Louis, M. (1999). High prevalence and incidence of sexually transmitted diseases in urban adolescent females despite moderate risk behaviors. *Journal of Infectious Diseases 180*(5), 1624-1631.

31. Boyer, C. B., Tschann, J. M., & Shafer, M. A. (1999). Predictors of risk for sexually transmitted diseases in ninth grade urban high school students. Journal of *Adolescent Research, 14*(4), 448-465.
32. Charron-Prochownik, D., Sereika, S. M., Becker, D., Jacober, S., Mansfield, J., White, N. H., & Trail, L. (2001). Reproductive health beliefs and behaviors in teens with diabetes: Application of the Expanded Health Belief Model. *Pediatric Diabetes,* 2(1), 30-39.
33. Barakat, L.P., Patterson, C.A., Daniel, L.C., & Dampier, C. (2008). Quality of life among adolescents with sickle cell disease: Mediation of pain by internalizing symptoms and parenting stress. *Health and Quality of Life Outcomes,* 6(1), 60.
34. Mahavarkar, S. H., Madhu, C. K., & Mule, V. D. (2008). A comparative study of teenage pregnancy. *Journal of Obstetrics & Gynecology, 28*(6), 604-607.
35. Alford, S., Huberman, B., Moss, T., & Hauser, D. (2003). Science and success: Sex education and other programs that work to prevent teen pregnancy HIV and sexually transmitted infections.
36. Ickovics, J. R., Niccolai, L. M., Lewis, J. B., Kershaw, T. S., & Ethier, K. A. (2003). High postpartum rates of sexually transmitted infections among teens: Pregnancy as a window of opportunity for prevention. *Sexually Transmitted Infections, 79*(6), 469-473.
37. Adimora, A. A., & Schoenbach, V. J. (2005). Social context, sexual networks, and racial disparities in rates of sexually transmitted infections. *Journal of Infectious Diseases, 191*(Supplement 1), S115-S122.
38. Zimet, G. D., Mays, R. M., & Fortenberry, D. J. (2000). Vaccines against sexually transmitted infections: promise and problems of the magic bullets for prevention and control. *Sexually Transmitted Diseases,* 27(1), 49-52.
39. Sellers, D. E., McGraw, S. A., & McKinlay, J. B. (1994). Does the promotion and distribution of condoms increase teen

sexual activity? Evidence from an HIV prevention program for Latino youth. *American Journal of Public Health, 84*(12), 1952-1959.

40. Terry, A., Szabo, A., & Griffiths, M. (2004). The exercise addiction inventory: A new brief screening tool. *Addiction Research and Theory, 12*(5), 489-499.

41. Long, C., & Smith, J. (1990). Treatment of compulsive over-exercising in anorexia nervosa: A case study. *Behavioural Psychotherapy, 18*(4), 295-306.

42. Davis, C., Kennedy, S. H., Ralevski, E., Dionne, M., Brewer, H., Neitzert, C., & Ratusny, D. (1995). Obsessive compulsiveness and physical activity in anorexia nervosa and high-level exercising. *Journal of Psychosomatic Research, 39*(8), 967-976.

43. Bamber, D., Cockerill, I. M., & Carroll, D. (2000). The pathological status of exercise dependence. *British Journal of Sports Medicine, 34*(2), 125-132.

44. Hughes, T. L., & Eliason, M. (2002). Substance use and abuse in lesbian, gay, bisexual and transgender populations. *Journal of Primary Prevention, 22*(3), 263-298.

45. Boehmer, U. (2002). Twenty years of public health research: Inclusion of lesbian, gay, bisexual, and transgender populations. *American Journal of Public Health, 92*(7), 1125-1130.

46. Gates, G. J. (2011). How many people are lesbian, gay, bisexual and transgender?

47. Conron, K. J., Scott, G., Stowell, G. S., & Landers, S. J. (2012). Transgender health in Massachusetts: Results from a household probability sample of adults. *American Journal of Public Health, 102*(1), 118-122.

48. Garofalo, R., Wolf, R.C., Wissow, L.S., et al. (1999). Sexual orientation and risk of suicide attempts among a representative sample of youth. *Archives of Pediatrics and Adolescent Medicine, 153*(5), 487-93.

49. Conron, K.J., Mimiaga, M.J., & Landers, S.J. (2010). A population-based study of sexual orientation identity and gender differences in adult health. *American Journal of Public Health, 100*(10), 1953-60.

50. Xavier, J., Honnold, J., & Bradford, J. (2007). The health, health-related needs, and lifecourse experiences of transgender Virginians. Virginia HIV Community Planning Committee and Virginia Department of Health. Richmond, VA.
51. National Gay and Lesbian Taskforce. (2009). National transgender discrimination survey: Preliminary findings. Washington, DC.
52. Newman, A. (2001). Adolescent consent to routine medical and surgical treatment: A proposal to simplify the law of teenage medical decision-making. *Journal of Legal Medicine, 22*(4), 501-532.
53. Jacobson, L. D., & Wilkinson, C. E. (1994). Review of teenage health: time for a new direction. *The British Journal of General Practice, 44*(386), 420.
54. Marks, A., Malizio, J., Hoch, J. et al. (1983). Assessment of health needs and willingness to utilize health care resources of adolescents in a suburban population. *Journal of Pediatrics, 102*, 456-460.
55. Beach, S. R., Brody, G. H., Lei, M. K., Gibbons, F. X., Gerrard, M., Simons, R. L., & Philibert, R. A. (2013). Impact of child sex abuse on adult psychopathology: A genetically and epigenetically informed investigation. *Journal of Family Psychology, 27*(1), 3.
56. Runyan, D., Wattam, C., Ikeda, R., Hassan, F., Ramiro, L., Camara, V. D.,... & Raymonville, M. (2013). Child abuse and neglect by parents and other caregivers. DST--*Jornal Brasileiro de Doenã § as Sexualmente Transmissãveis, 15*(3), 57-86.
57. MacMillan, H. L., Tanaka, M., Duku, E., Vaillancourt, T., & Boyle, M. H. (2013). Child physical and sexual abuse in a community sample of young adults: Results from the Ontario Child Health Study. *Child Abuse & Neglect, 37*(1), 14-21.
58. Schwartz, W. (2001). Closing the Achievement Gap: Principles for Improving the Educational Success of All Students. ERIC Digest.

59. Crosby, R. A., DiClemente, R. J., Wingood, G. M., Cobb, B. K., Harrington, K., Davies, S. L.,... & Oh, M. K. (2001). HIV/STD-protective benefits of living with mothers in perceived supportive families: a study of high-risk African American female teens. *Preventive Medicine, 33*(3), 175-178.
60. Rotheram-Borus, M. J., Lee, M. B., Murphy, D. A., Futterman, D., Duan, N., Birnbaum, J. M., & Teens Linked to Care Consortium. (2001). Efficacy of a preventive intervention for youths living with HIV. *American Journal of Public Health, 91*(3), 400.
61. Ferris, M., Burau, K., Schweitzer, A. M., Mihale, S., Murray, N., Preda, A., & Kline, M. (2007). The influence of disclosure of HIV diagnosis on time to disease progression in a cohort of Romanian children and teens. *AIDS Care, 19*(9), 1088-1094.
62. Hoppe, M. J., Graham, L., Wilsdon, A., Wells, E. A., Nahom, D., & Morrison, D. M. (2004). Teens speak out about HIV/AIDS: focus group discussions about risk and decision-making. *Journal of Adolescent Health, 35*(4), 345-e27.
63. Crosby, R. A., DiClemente, R. J., Wingood, G. M., & Harrington, K. (2002). HIV/STD prevention benefits of living in supportive families: A prospective analysis of high risk African-American female teens. *American Journal of Health Promotion, 16*(3), 142-145.
64. Bray, G. A., Nielsen, S. J., & Popkin, B. M. (2004). Consumption of high-fructose corn syrup in beverages may play a role in the epidemic of obesity. *The American Journal of Clinical Nutrition, 79*(4), 537-543.
65. Tordoff, M. G., & Alleva, A. M. (1990). Effect of drinking soda sweetened with aspartame or high-fructose corn syrup on food intake and body weight. *The American Journal of Clinical Nutrition, 51*(6), 963-969.
66. White, J. S. (2008). Straight talk about high-fructose corn syrup: what it is and what it ain't. *The American Journal of Clinical Nutrition*.

INDEX

A

abstinence 83, 84
abuse 12, 113, 116, 119, 132, 133, 146, 150, 157, 158, 161, 162, 163, 164, 168, 171, 183, 201, 221, 222
acne 62, 63, 67, 68, 86, 100, 102, 156
addiction 39, 42, 43, 44, 161, 164, 165, 167, 201, 221
AIDS 60, 74, 77, 223
alcohol 36, 50, 80, 82, 103, 116, 150, 155, 156, 161, 167, 173, 175, 176, 178, 179, 192
antiperspirant 69
asthma 87, 93, 94, 95, 96, 97, 167

B

body mass index 88, 89, 93, 210, 217
bullying 92, 110, 113, 114, 118, 120, 121, 125, 133, 139, 140, 141, 142, 182, 185

C

caloric intake 16, 92
carbohydrate 23
carbohydrates 15, 16, 22, 23, 24, 25, 42, 102
communication 52, 108, 112, 121, 126, 136, 184
condom 78, 79, 80
contraception 78, 80, 82, 85, 203

D

deodorant 69
depression 12, 19, 43, 49, 73, 138, 153, 155, 182, 183, 186, 191, 194, 218
diabetes 27, 39, 56, 57, 87, 97, 98, 99, 100, 156, 206, 209, 211, 220
diet 13, 14, 15, 21, 22, 24, 26, 28, 31, 32, 33, 36, 49, 54, 71, 74, 89, 101, 102
disease 13, 31, 56, 59, 73, 74, 75, 76, 77, 80, 83, 86, 96, 97, 99, 103, 167, 211, 219, 220, 223
drugs 33, 77, 80, 82, 83, 102, 103, 113, 114, 116, 132, 141, 144, 150, 155, 156, 158, 159, 160, 161, 163, 164, 169, 171, 172, 175, 185, 192, 201
DUI 177

E

eating disorders 19, 20, 43, 56, 155, 205
estrogen 14, 61, 64
exercise 13, 30, 35, 36, 37, 38, 39, 40, 41, 42, 43, 44, 45, 46, 54, 95, 96, 98, 103, 192, 206, 221
extracurricular activities 50
eye 56, 57, 130

F

Facebook 123, 124, 180
family 11, 31, 50, 55, 57, 63, 71, 76, 77, 91, 99, 110, 111, 114, 118, 120, 123, 128, 144, 149, 157, 158, 161, 162, 165, 175, 180, 184, 185, 189, 192, 193, 196, 197, 199
fats 14, 16, 22, 23, 29, 30, 31, 32, 33, 92
friends 111, 138

H

hair 11, 62, 63, 67, 69, 70, 84, 101
health insurance 117
heterosexual 114, 115
HIV 60, 74, 75, 76, 77, 78, 85, 117, 163, 201, 220, 221, 222, 223
homosexual 114, 116
hormones 16, 30, 39, 61, 64, 66, 102, 155, 161, 183
hygiene 56, 58, 66, 69, 85, 99, 102

I

infertility 71, 72, 85
insulin 25, 26, 27, 39, 97, 98, 156

J

junk food 22, 30, 155

L

LGBT 105, 113, 115, 116, 117, 119, 120, 121
lipids 16, 29, 30, 31

M

macronutrients 18
meditation 103, 185, 187, 188, 189
menstruation 64, 65
metabolism 18, 21, 25, 26, 28, 30, 31, 39, 40, 92
micronutrients 18

N

nicotine 103, 165, 167
nutrients 13, 17, 18, 22, 30, 92, 99
nutrition 13, 29, 92, 103, 155, 205, 206, 207, 208, 210, 211, 212, 213

O

obesity 19, 21, 27, 29, 30, 31, 39, 88, 89, 90, 92, 98, 104, 155, 210, 211, 212, 213, 223

P

parents 5, 11, 72, 92, 93, 108, 109, 110, 111, 118, 119, 139, 140, 142, 143, 145, 146, 147, 149, 153, 157, 165, 173, 182, 184, 185, 186, 196, 199, 200, 201, 202, 203, 208, 212, 222
peer pressure 111, 139, 163, 164
pregnancy 64, 72, 73, 74, 78, 79, 80, 81, 82, 83, 85, 102, 133, 151, 159, 199, 200, 201, 217, 218, 219, 220
proteins 14, 22, 40, 50
puberty 13, 61, 63, 64, 66, 67, 68, 69, 100, 101, 102, 104

R

respect 110, 135, 141, 143, 144, 145, 146, 149, 186, 190, 195
responsibility 72, 104, 105, 146, 147, 148, 149, 151, 190, 193, 195, 199, 201

S

sexual intercourse 82
sexually transmitted diseases 77, 82, 85, 159, 168, 201, 202, 219, 220
sexually transmitted infections 78, 117, 133, 151, 163, 220
sexual orientation 113, 115, 117, 201, 221
shaving 70
sleep 44, 49, 51, 52, 53, 54, 130, 183
social media 36, 52, 122, 123, 126, 128, 130, 131
stress 41, 42, 43, 45, 49, 50, 84, 91, 100, 103, 107, 120, 152, 153, 154, 155, 165, 183, 187, 198, 208, 218, 220
sugar 21, 23, 25, 28, 50, 54, 92, 97, 98, 99, 100, 102, 156
suicide 53, 73, 113, 114, 116, 118, 124, 125, 133, 156, 180, 181, 182, 183, 184, 185, 217, 218, 221

T

teeth 18, 58, 59
tobacco 58, 116, 155, 156, 164, 165, 166, 167
trans fats 31
transgender 114, 115, 116, 221, 222

U

unhealthy relationship 132, 136

W

water 21, 23, 24, 33, 34, 35, 36, 43, 54, 70, 99, 119, 120, 134, 166, 218, 219

ABOUT THE AUTHOR

Antwala Robinson, DNP, FNP-BC, APRN - "The Wellness Agent™" is an authority and agent of change to those looking to live a life of total well-being and create their own destiny. She holds a doctor of nursing practice degree, is a board-certified family nurse practitioner, and is licensed as an advanced practice registered nurse. Antwala has over 19 years' experience as a primary care provider, nurse, educator, researcher, trainer, speaker, health and life coach, author, and consultant. She is a mentor for Communities In Schools, "the nation's leading community-based organization that helps kids succeed in school and prepare for life." Antwala is passionate about health and wellness, and is on a personal crusade to help people of all ages worldwide to take charge of their health and life. She resides in Atlanta, GA, with her teenage daughter.

www.ingramcontent.com/pod-product-compliance
Lightning Source LLC
Chambersburg PA
CBHW051942290426
44110CB00015B/2080